Toxicology: What Everyone Should Know

Toxicology: What Everyone Should Know

A Book for Researchers, Consumers, Journalists and Politicians

Aalt Bast

Jaap C. Hanekamp

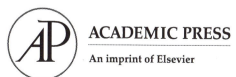

ACADEMIC PRESS

An imprint of Elsevier

Academic Press is an imprint of Elsevier
125 London Wall, London EC2Y 5AS, United Kingdom
525 B Street, Suite 1800, San Diego, CA 92101-4495, United States
50 Hampshire Street, 5th Floor, Cambridge, MA 02139, United States
The Boulevard, Langford Lane, Kidlington, Oxford OX5 1GB, United Kingdom

Notices
Knowledge and best practice in this field are constantly changing. As new research and experience broaden
our understanding, changes in research methods, professional practices, or medical treatment may become
necessary.

Practitioners and researchers must always rely on their own experience and knowledge in evaluating and
using any information, methods, compounds, or experiments described herein. In using such information or
methods they should be mindful of their own safety and the safety of others, including parties for whom they
have a professional responsibility.

To the fullest extent of the law, neither the Publisher nor the authors, contributors, or editors, assume any
liability for any injury and/or damage to persons or property as a matter of products liability, negligence or
otherwise, or from any use or operation of any methods, products, instructions, or ideas contained in the
material herein.

British Library Cataloguing-in-Publication Data
A catalogue record for this book is available from the British Library

Library of Congress Cataloging-in-Publication Data
A catalog record for this book is available from the Library of Congress

ISBN: 978-0-12-805348-5

For Information on all Academic Press publications
visit our website at https://www.elsevier.com/books-and-journals

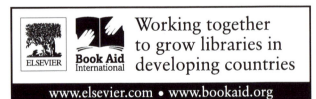

Working together
to grow libraries in
developing countries

www.elsevier.com • www.bookaid.org

Publisher: Mica Haley
Acquisition Editor: Erin Hill-Parks
Editorial Project Manager: Tracy Tufaga
Production Project Manager: Kirsty Halterman and Karen East
Cover Designer: Christian Bilbow

Typeset by MPS Limited, Chennai, India

Contents

Preface

The book before you is an expression of both author's knowledge and understanding of and great enthusiasm for toxicology. To be sure, books abound on this subject in all sorts of shapes and sizes. What we tried to do here is arrange the central themes in a text that should appeal to all and sundry with an interest to match our own. Students may find in our book a solid basis for master studies and research, and even an undergraduate could muster different aspects of our text without difficulty. Journalists would be able to contextualize the next iteration of "healthy diets" or the dangers of certain chemicals in our direct environment. The general public that sometimes feels threatened by the chemical world we all live in might find reassurance but also proper warning that carries the scientific basis known for centuries and the newest insights that could change our understanding of "the toxic."

We specifically aimed for a concise text without the usual jargon that might baffle most readers. Surely, we have failed at some level to completely eradicate the science-speak so typical for the halls of academia. But, not all language can be so "purified" as specific words and terms identify very particular topics that we tried, as best we could, to explicate to the reader. In all this we should keep in mind that no matter how complex certain toxicological subjects are, they are still fundamentally embedded in everyday life. Exposure to "the chemical," with all that entails, is an everyday experience that is encapsulated by every breath we take, every lunch, dinner, or breakfast we consume, and every glass of wine (or whisky) we enjoy. All that knowledge could not be contained in the biggest library in the world or even all libraries combined. For that reason we limited ourselves to some 100 odd pages, heeding the words of Blaise Pascal, the famous French mathematician, physicist, writer, and Christian philosopher, who once noted that one of his many letters was "very long, simply because I had no leisure to make it shorter." We have taken that "leisure" at heart and tried painstakingly not to be wordy, boring, or otherwise pedantic. We sincerely hope the reader agrees.

Aalt Bast and Jaap C. Hanekamp
May 2017
The Netherlands

Chapter 1

From Pretaster to Toxicologist

In the milk scandal in 2008 in China, water was added to raw milk to increase its volume so more that it could be sold as the real deal. This dilution obviously results in a lower protein concentration. The protein level of milk is usually checked through measuring the nitrogen content of the milk. By adding nitrogen containing melamine to the diluted milk and the powdered infant formula the nitrogen content increases and thereby the apparent protein content. Melamine is widely used as a base material for plastics used in dishware and adhesives. The ingestion of melamine leads to kidney failure; symptoms are irritability, blood in urine, little or no urine, high blood pressure, and eventually death. The use of melamine killed six babies and made 300,000 ill. Widespread reports indicated that senior Chinese officials knew about the contamination but suppressed it because of fears of bad publicity. A dairy farmer and milk production center manager were convicted for the scandal and executed in 2009. Several others were sentenced to jail.

TOXIC DANGERS FOR ANCIENT MAN AND PHARAOS

Toxicology is without doubt the oldest scientific discipline. Ancient man collected food and had to have the knowledge of what could be eaten safely. Plants cannot run away and to safeguard their existence they have thorns, a bitter taste, and they contain a wide variety of toxins (also known as phytotoxins) to protect themselves against herbivores. It has been estimated that 99.99% (by weight) of our intake of pesticides through food is of natural origin. Plants make their own pesticides. This is perhaps the biggest discovery in the field of toxicology ever made, even before this field came into being as we know it today. The world is full of chemicals, and some of them we respond to in less than fortuitous ways. That we have understood since the dawn of time.

Ancient people were plant collectors and their mere survival depended on extensive knowledge on plants toxicities. The question which plants could be consumed safely probably was continuously boggling their minds.

Over centuries we have been able to improve plants in such a way that the toxins present in plants were reduced, thus making them more suitable for human consumption. Examples of natural pesticides in foods are however still easily given. The most discussed agricultural crop family is the

Toxicology: What Everyone Should Know. DOI: http://dx.doi.org/10.1016/B978-0-12-805348-5.00001-6

Solanaceae, or nightshades, which includes the potato, tomato, and eggplant (aubergine). These crop plants synthesize several so-called alkaloids such as chaconine and solanine found in the potato and giving it a bitter taste especially when green, and tomatine found in, unsurprisingly, tomatoes. These and other alkaloids possess powerful insecticidal and fungicidal properties, although some insect species have adapted. And, these potato chemicals are certainly not harmless to us. In potato breeding, for instance, one should be always be wary of the ability of new cultivars to produce toxic levels of alkaloids.

The classic case demonstrating this is the Lenape cultivar produced in the 1960s. This then-new potato had good insect resistance and a high solids content, both desirable characteristics especially for the production of potato chips. However, illness after ingestion of this potato was reported on a number of occasions, such as nausea and vomiting. It was later determined that Lenape had very high levels of alkaloids, and the variety was never released for widespread commercial use as it was too toxic.

Many spices prized for their taste are known to have many different chemicals that act as repellents against all sorts of organisms. Safrole, an effective pesticide, is found in nutmeg and black pepper. Safrole is known to be toxic to the liver and might even induce cancer.

Or what about mustard and wasabi and their burning taste loved by many (including us). Allyl isothiocyanate, also known as mustard oil, is the culprit here. The compound is a plant-defense chemical against herbivores (such as horses, deer, and cows). It makes plants that produce such spicy-tasting chemicals unattractive to plant-eating animals.

Wasabi is traditionally eaten with sushi in the Japanese cuisine. One reason offered for this custom, apart from the acquired taste, is that allyl isothiocyanate suppresses bacterial growth. Thereby, wasabi makes the consumption of raw fish safer. To be sure, wasabi might not be agreeable to some, and should not be consumed in large quantities. Wasabi paste is meant to be mixed with soy sauce and used only in very small amounts.

The food we eat is thus characterized by all sorts of chemicals that either predominates taste—allyl isothiocyanate in wasabi—or are inadvertently part and parcel of the consumable alkaloids in potatoes. So the good and the bad, if such a distinction can be made straightforwardly, are intertwined in the total diet we consume every day. Sometimes, however, accidents occur which makes us realize that the original plant was a strongly toxic species.

In 2015 it was reported that a German pensioner was killed by eating a courgette stew. The courgettes were home grown. Apparently the stew tasted bitter but the man and his wife ate it despite its taste. They were unaware of the bitter toxins hidden in the plant. The couple was hospitalized and diagnosed with severe poisoning. The wife recovered but the husband died.

The toxic substance with the bitter taste belong to the group of cucurbitacins. The basic structure of these bitter-tasting compounds is given in

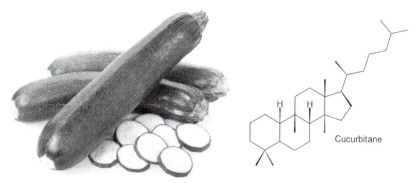

FIGURE 1.1   Picture of courgettes and chemical structure of cucurbitane in the courgettes.

Fig. 1.1. These natural toxins are founds in plants of the Cucurbitaceae family as pumpkins and gourds such as courgettes. The cucurbitacins have been bred out of commercially sold seeds. Gourds growing next to ornamental breeds of pumpkins can be dangerous because cross-pollination may infect edible varieties and seeds from previous years may become hazardous.

Also molds that grow on crops can produce strong toxins. The fungus *Aspergillus*, with the most notable ones being *Aspergillus flavus* and *Aspergillus parasiticus,* grows on among others peanuts, corn, or pistachio nuts. The mycotoxins produced by *Aspergillus* are called aflatoxins. These compounds are toxic and belong to the most carcinogenic substances known. After entering the body, aflatoxins are metabolized by the liver to very reactive break down products which are either detoxified by subsequent reactions in the liver or they bind to DNA in the liver and cause cancer. The color of the several aflatoxins is blueish or greenish. It therefore does not come as a surprise that many toxicologists and chemists are reluctant to eat pistachio nuts (Fig. 1.2).

During humid periods ergot fungi of the genus *Claviceps* grow on rye and other cereals. The prominent member is *Claviceps purpurea*. The ergot replaces the grain of the rye in dark purplish kernels. Eating bread-containing flour made from grains holding ergot may lead to severe toxicity. This is called ergotism and causes hallucinations and convulsions. The vaso-constrictions by the ergot alkaloids (the toxic compounds from the ergot) lead to a burning pain and was called Saint Anthony's Fire and eventually give gangrene (dying tissue of the toes, feet, and fingers). Also diarrhea, itching, mania or psychosis, headache, nausea, and vomiting may occur after eating the infected rye bread. During the Middle Ages, the regularly occurring dancing mania have been ascribed to ergot poisoning. Several paintings from those days show these mass hysteric dancings of large groups of people. The ergot alkaloids can also be passed from mother to child via lactation (Fig. 1.3).

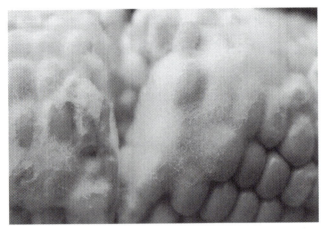

FIGURE 1.2   Picture of molded corn.

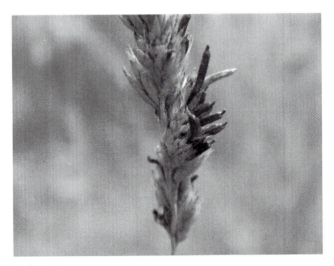

FIGURE 1.3   Infected rye.

These poisonous molds are not only dangerous to us. Regularly there are reports on seemingly mysterious deaths of cows. Sometimes viral infections like the infectious bovine rhinotracheitis or the bovine virus diarrhea are pinpointed as the cause of death. But the 200 cows that suddenly died in 2011 in Wisconsin were poisoned by eating spoiled sweet potatoes. The potatoes were not suitable for human consumption anymore and were therefore fed to the cows. The mold growing on the potatoes was determined to be *Fusarium solani*. Ingestion of these infested potatoes gives exposure to the pneumotoxin 4-ipomeanol. The clinical pathological picture is indistinguishable from

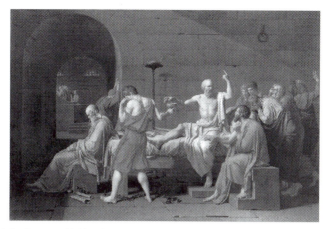

FIGURE 1.4   Socrates drinking from the beaker, surrounded by youth.

acute bovine pulmonary emphysema and edema. Similar cases on rotten sweet potatoes triggering cow deaths have been documented in 2001, 2003, and 2007.

Besides these unintended intoxications via our food, planned suicides, executions, or murders may also occur via the food. Famous is the story of the Greek philosopher Socrates who was punished for both spreading his "radical ideas" to the youth of Athens and of impiety via drinking an extract of hemlock (Fig. 1.4).

Emperors, kings, and pharaohs had pretasters to protect them from intoxications. Their lives were always in danger and the food was tested before they took the food themselves. One of the earliest written stories about pretasters can be found in the Bible (Genesis 40). Joseph met the cupbearer and baker of the king of Egypt who apparently committed an offense against their lord and king of Egypt. Both the cupbearer and the baker had dreams, and Joseph who saw their downcast faces interpreted on their request, their dreams. To the cupbearer Joseph said that he would be restored to his office and would place Pharaoh's cup in his hands as formerly. The interpretation of the chief baker's dream was less favorable because it was predicted that he would be hanged on a tree.

And indeed, three days later at the Pharaoh's birthday (Genesis 40:21−22): He [the Pharaoh (authors)] restored the chief cupbearer to his position, and he placed the cup in Pharaoh's hand. But he hanged the chief baker, as Joseph had interpreted to them.

The chief cupbearer and baker presumably were the pretasters of the Pharaoh. In fact they were high priests, important persons within the religious circles and of high social status. You might compare them with modern toxicologists. The importance and high social status might underline that [smile (authors)]. However, the hanging scene makes the comparison less attractive of course.

Also in recent times political poisonings take place. During his campaign for president in Ukraine in 2004 Viktor Yushchenko was poisoned with dioxin. The disfiguring cloracne in his face is a characteristic symptom of dioxin poisoning. Dioxins are a group of chlorinated molecules. They are formed as by-product in waste incineration. The most toxic dioxin is 2,3,7,8-tetrachlorodibenzo-*p*-dioxin abbreviated as TCDD. In 1976 a small chemical manufacturing plant exploded in Seveso (approximately 25 km north from Milan in north Italy) generated and released dioxins and the residential population was exposed to it. The exposed Italian children showed the same skin damage as observed with Yushchenko.

SWITCHING FUNCTIONALITY: FROM NATURAL TOXINS TO DRUGS

Ancient discoveries frequently resulted from accidents. A nice example is the use of curare by Indian tribes in South America. The plant *Chodondendron tomentosum* and other plants of the rainforest were used to prepare an extract they called curare (the Indian word meaning poison). Arrow tips were submerged in the extract and used for hunting. The poison contained various components like d-tubocurarine. This compound blocks the signal transduction from nerves to skeletal muscles by binding to the receptor that usually reacts with the normal nerve transmitter acetylcholine. This inhibits the contraction of the muscle and the hunted animal can be caught. A high dose can even block the respiratory muscles of the animal and leads to its death. After that, the paralyzed prey can be safely consumed because the uptake of curare from the gastro-intestinal tract is limited and its excretion overwhelms the effect of the toxin.

d-Tubocurarine was used in treating muscle spasms and in anesthesia, if complete immobilization was needed during delicate surgery. Anesthetists have now new analogs of d-tubocurarine at their disposal that are safer to use.

The most common drug known by everyone is aspirin. This was in fact originally a trade name of the compound acetylsalicylic acid by the company Bayer AG. Aspirin became popular in the first half of the 20th century. The American patent held by Bayer expired in 1917, which led to a proliferation of aspirin products.

The idea of synthesizing acetylsalicylic acid came from the historic use of salicylic acid. This substance was originally obtained from the willow tree (Latin: *salix*). Salicylic acid was known easing pains and reducing fevers. For that reason the bark of the willow tree has been used for many centuries over the globe by Native Americans, Europeans, Chinese, ancient Greeks, and Egyptians.

The earlier mentioned ergot alkaloids from the ergot fungus contain lysergic acid. This compound has been used to synthesize LSD, the abbreviation of lysergic acid diethylamide in 1938. It has hallucinogenic properties and has been used by psychiatrists in the previous century to investigate schizophrenia. LSD is frequently indicated as "acid" and has been used extensively in the "flower power" period in the 1960s. Sometimes it was mixed through lemonade at parties through which ignorant partygoers were caught by strong visual "trips." It has been visualized quite poignantly in Terry Gilliam's *Fear and Loathing in Las Vegas* (Fig. 1.5).

Early pharmacists possessed a broad knowledge on botany. Many medications derived from plants and studies of the Materia Medica were a necessity. Seminal examples include plants like the *Digitalis purpura*, known as foxglove. The plant is regarded as extremely toxic because of the presence of digoxine. Administered in the right dose it is used as a drug in the treatment of heart failure. It increases the beating force of the heart. Moreover, it is used in the treatment of certain forms of irregular heart beat (atrium fibrillation) and still has a very important place in the pharmacotherapy in cardiology. This compound has a small therapeutic window, that is the difference between the concentration needed for an effect and the toxic concentration is very narrow. The blood plasma level should be between 0.8 and 2.0 ng/mL.

Many antitumor agents are derived from plants and used directly or chemically modified to enhance their activity and to sometimes lower their side effects. In a search for new cytostatics a screening program of plant extracts was initiated by the National Cancer Institute in the USA. It was found that the extract of *Taxus brevifolia* was active against several tumor cells. The isolated active compound from the extract mixture was paclitaxel which appeared to be active against ovarium carcinoma. From 2013 a

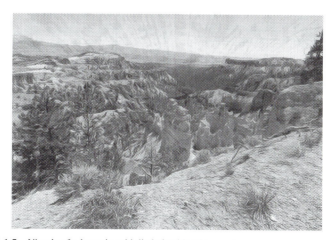

FIGURE 1.5   Visuals of a lysergic acid diethylamide trip experience.

semisynthetic method has been developed to make paclitaxel from *Taxus baccata*. Also plant cell fermentation processes have been employed using a *Taxus* cell line to make paclitaxel.

Doxorubicin is an anthracycline antibiotic with oncolytic (antitumor) activity. It is a very effective antitumor agent isolated from the bacteria *Streptomyces peucetius*. It inhibits the growth of rapidly dividing cells and it is widely used among others in the treatment of acute lymphatic leukemia and mamma and ovarium carcinoma. Doxorubicin has various long-term side effects that particularly manifest at higher dosages. Doxorubicin-induced heart toxicity has been investigated quite extensively because after surviving the cancer, the quality of life might be hampered by this toxicity. Many derivatives of doxorubicin have been synthesized over several decades, but it still plays a prominent role in oncology.

Many antibiotics are isolated from molds. Probably the most notable example is the discovery of penicillin by the Scottish scientist Alexander Fleming in 1928. He was working on staphylococci, bacteria, which can cause infections. On one of his Petri disks he discerned a mold, *Penicillium notatum*, and noticed that the staphylococci around that mold disappeared. It appeared that this mold was able to secrete a bacteria killing compound, which he called penicillin. Later research learned that the antibiotic blocks the building of the cellular membrane of bacteria. It started the era of antibiotics.

TOXICOLOGISTS IN CLINIC, NUTRITION, ENVIRONMENT, AND FORENSICS

A toxicologist tries to understand (and thereby predict) the effect of compounds on life forms. Toxicology encompasses environmental, clinical, nutritional, and forensic toxicology.

Every handbook on toxicology begins with citing the adage of Paracelsus (1493–1541): "(in Latin) *Sola dosis facit venenum*," the dose makes the poison. His real name was Philippus Aureolus Theophrastus Bombastus von Hohenheim. It is suggested that the use of pompous, exaggerated phrases or words are said to be bombastic because it is reminiscent to the way of writing and speaking of this "Bombastus" von Hohenheim. Because he regarded his thoughts further reaching than those of Aulus Cornelius Celsus, a famous Roman physician of the 1st century, he used the name Paracelsus (against Celsus). Another explanation for the name Paracelsus was that it is the Latin form of the German name Hohenheim: *Para* (Greek) meaning after or from and *celsus* (Latin) meaning haughty, arrogant, and proud.

Paracelsus was a German Swiss physician, philosopher, theologian, botanist, and astrologer. His realization that everything is toxic and that only the dose determines whether the toxicity is observed still forms the basic principle of toxicology. Paracelsus treated syphilis with arsenic and apparently had good results in using a relatively low dose. However, at higher dose not only the syphilis was gone but also the patient was lost. A striking observation illustrating his notion that too much of a compound (a high dose) always leads to toxicity. He is credited the founder of the toxicology.

The history of toxicology goes back even further. Documents from China have been found from 2700 BC in which toxins from plants and fishes have been described. Preparation and administration of more than 800 drugs and poisons are found in Egyptian writings of 1900–1200 BC. From Hindu-Indian notes on toxins and antidotes are known from 800 BC Greek physicians classified more than 600 plant, animal, and mineral toxins during the 1st century. Romans (50–400 AC) also knew how to use poisons for murders and executions.

Avicenna (or Ibn Sina) who lived from 980 to 1037 was an Islamic physician (physicist, philosopher, and alchemist) of Persian origin and an authority in the field of toxins and protective agents against toxins. In 1280 the Spanish rabbi Maimonides wrote a first aid book on intoxications. He was also known by the name Rambam (the acronym of his full Hebrew name). He produced an impressive body of work. The Dutch expression "you worked like rambam" entails that you worked very hard and were very productive. Many schools and hospitals across the globe are named after Maimonides.

Nowadays we trust that the food we buy is not contaminated with toxins from bacteria or molds, and that the endogenous toxins are low enough not to harm us directly. Governmental agencies like the American Food and Drug Administration and the European Food Safety Authority are established to safeguard our food.

We rely on cooks for the preparation of risky food, like the Fugu fish, a Japanese delicacy. The fish contains a toxin (viz. tetrodotoxin) which can be found in ovaries and liver. Japanese cooks need special skills and are trained to safely prepare the fish. Nevertheless each year several people die by eating one of the Japanese favorites.

Historic awareness already unfolded an extensive field of the so-called nutritional toxicology. Recent developments will further emphasize this field. Since, during the last decades, the so-called Novel Foods entered the market. Novel Foods are foods which have never been eaten by the consumer before. Especially the EU lately developed the Novel Food Regulation. The new food ingredients or products should not present a risk to public health, should not be nutritionally disadvantageous when replacing a similar food, should not be misleading to the consumer, and must undergo a scientific assessment prior to authorization to ensure safety.

Other toxicological disciplines emerged after the Industrial Revolution. In the field of occupation toxicology much improved. One of the first reports in this area is the discovery by the British surgeon Sir Percival Pott (1714–1780). He discovered that boys who worked in London as chimney sweepers got scrotum cancer. Pott associated the exposure to soot to "chimney sweeps carcinoma." Now we know that the environmental carcinogen benzo[a]pyrene in soot is responsible for the occurrence of cancer.

Also think about the miners who were exposed to mine dust over several years and as a result of that could get pneumoconiosis, an inflammatory disease of the lungs, with frequently devastating consequences.

In the twenties of the previous century, a well-paid job was painting the numerals and hands of clocks and watches with radium. The radioactive radium gave beautiful light and made the clock hands nicely visible. Positioned in long rows in big halls, young women minutely painted the dials. With the lips a sharp tip was produced to the brush to assist the painting. Exposure to radioactive radium led to rarely occurring malignancies.

Environmental toxicology studies the effect of chemical or biological agents on living organisms and ecosystems. The book entitled "Silent Spring," by Rachel Carson in 1962 was an indictment of the rampant use of pesticides and the poorly regulated emissions of chemical waste (see Chapter 4: Nature Knows Best—Chemicals From the Geobiological Sphere).

The clinical toxicologist is frequently originally trained as a pharmacist. Intentional or unintentional overdose is the field of interest. With the older growing population frequent examples of poly-pharmacy occur. Elderly people take many drugs. These prescribed drugs are sometimes combined with over-the-counter medication. Unexpected interactions can easily occur and in fact it is estimated that about 20% of the hospitalizations of elderly patients can be ascribed to wrong use of medication (see Chapter 3: The Coping Body—A Myriad of Exposures).

If the mechanism of the toxic drug response is understood a proper treatment can be proposed. Things change when a specific patient reacts to a drug in an unexpected negative manner. This so-called idiosyncratic toxicity can be very severe and the treatment will be less clear. The cause for this type of toxicity may be the genetic background or the diet or the specific combination of drugs of this specific person. It can pose a real puzzle for the clinical toxicologist.

The enigmatic puzzles to which forensic toxicologist is subjected appeals to the imagination. Watching TV series like *CSI, NCIS, Law and Order*, or *Bones* makes you believe that forensic toxicological problems are solved within an hour (i.e., including the commercials). In reality it takes several weeks and the work will undoubtedly not always be successful.

Testing for doping in sport belongs to the work area of the forensic toxicologist. A striking example in this respect is the former East-German (DDR) female athlete Katrin Krabbe. She won several 100 m and 200 m titles. In 1992 she, and several of her teammates, was tested positive for the clenbuterol. This is clinically used as an antiasthma drug because it relaxes the smooth muscles of the lungs. These type of (so-called beta2 adrenergic receptor stimulating) drugs have also a positive influence on fat oxidation

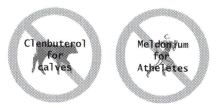

FIGURE 1.6 Examples of prohibited use of medication: Clenbuterol in calves and meldonium for athletes.

and muscle protein formation and thus have a stimulating effect on performance.

Clenbuterol has also been used illegally in calf rearing to get more and whiter meat (Fig. 1.6). Interestingly we also investigated newly developed beta2 adrenergic receptor stimulating agents. In those days we received a phone call of a pigeon fancier who requested some of the new compounds from the patent which indicated the impressive growth of the guinea pigs on which the compound was tested. The compound might assist his pigeons in winning races

Recently, the cardiac drug meldonium (trade name Meldronate) was in the news. Since January 2016 it is listed by the World Anti-Doping Agency. Several top athletes from former eastern bloc countries where it has been registered as a drug have been tested positive. Meldonium has not been registered in Western Europe and the USA. It is meant to increase the blood flow through the coronary arteries in cardiac patients. Public data on the performance-enhancing efficacy in healthy persons are however scarce.

Toxicology studies the properties of compounds and their effects on living organisms. The aim is to determine and understand their potential adverse effects in an attempt to protect human health. The scientific discipline has broadened and now also encompasses the preservation of the environment and plays a role in forensics as well.

REFERENCES AND FURTHER READING

Ames, B.N., Profet, M., Gold, L.S., 1990. Dietary pesticides (99.99% all natural). Proc. Natl. Acad. Sci. U.S.A. 87 (19), 7777−7781.

Bast, A., Haenen, G.R.M.M., Bruynzeel, A.M., van der Vijgh, W.J.F., 2007. Protection by flavonoids against anthracycline cardiotoxicity: from chemistry to clinical trials. Cardiovasc. Toxicol. 7 (2), 154−159.

Dambrova, M., Makrecka-Kuka, M., Vilskersts, R., Makarova, E., Kuka, J., Liepinsh, E., 2016. Pharmacological effects of meldonium: biochemical mechanisms and biomarkers of cardiometabolic activity. Pharmacol. Res. 113 (Pt B), 771−780.

⟨http://ec.europa.eu/food/safety/novel_food/legislation/index_en.htm⟩ (last accessed on June 13, 2016).

⟨http://www.huffingtonpost.com/2011/01/29/200-dead-cows-mystery-sol_n_815864.html⟩   (last accessed June 13, 2016).

⟨http://www.thelocal.de/20150821/courgette-stew-kills-pensioner-in-heidelberg⟩   (last accessed June 13, 2016).

⟨http://www.who.int/csr/media/faq/QAmelamine/en/⟩ (last accessed on June 13, 2016).

Chapter 2

Death by Dose—The Most Toxic Compounds

A fun night out? Let us go to an oxygen bar. A high concentration of oxygen gas (O_2) is bubbled through bottles containing aromatic flavors (e.g., mint or lavender) and led via small tubes hooked over the ears to openings under the nostrils where it is released. You are lured into the establishment because it is advertised that the blood oxygen concentration rises which will reduce stress, increase energy and alertness, and alleviates headaches. Recreational inhalation of oxygen: A fun night out, or an appropriate beginning of a chapter on "the most toxic compounds"?

THE CHEMISTRY OF OXYGEN

In this chapter we will focus on one of the most toxic compounds in our environment, oxygen (O_2). The struggles of its discovery, its role in evolution, and its reactivity will be looked at. We will show and explain the extreme toxicity of oxygen and its involvement in many age-related diseases. Questions on the possibilities to counteract its toxicity will be discussed. Finally we will show how, during evolution, we have been adapted to oxygen toxicity and how this adaptation process can still be used to benefit our health, adaptation being the keyword here.

The English theologian and chemist Joseph Priestley (1733−1804) is credited with the discovery of oxygen. He called the gas that he isolated "dephlostigated air," which he made by focusing sun rays on a sample of mercuric oxide. To his surprise mice survived in this "dephlostigated air." His ideas were in line with the prevailing idea that all burnable material comprised of two parts. One part was called phlogisticon which was given off when the substance containing it was burned. The residual part was thought to be the real form of the material.

As with many important discoveries, others at the same time had similar ideas. In fact the Swedish pharmacist Carl Wilhelm Scheele produced oxygen gas in 1772, two years earlier than Priestley. The Frenchman Lavoisier conducted quantitative combustion experiments using oxidation in a closed environment. He reached the conclusion that air consisted of gases,

Toxicology: What Everyone Should Know. DOI: http://dx.doi.org/10.1016/B978-0-12-805348-5.00002-8

"vital air" which is used for the combustion and for respiration and "lifeless air" or azote. The latter is still the word for nitrogen in French.

"Vital air" was renamed by Lavoisier in 1777 to oxygène. This name appeared to be wrong because Lavoisier believed that oxygen was part of all acids (*oxys* (Greek) means acid or sharp taste of acid and −*genes* (Greek) means producer, oxygen is then "acid producer").

Not only in the life of scientists with their experiments and theories of the 18th century the struggle with oxygen was clearly visible. Also in the development and organization of life on earth as a whole the fight with oxygen played a crucial role.

The estimated age of our earth is 4.6 billion (4.6×10^9) years. Intense solar radiation bombarded the surface of the earth at 3500 million ($= 3.5$ billion) years when anaerobic life began. Blue green algae in the oceans acquired the ability to use the process of photosynthesis which uses solar energy, water, and carbon dioxide releasing oxygen at 2500 million years ago. The biological appearance of oxygen is called the Great Oxygenation Event. Obligate anaerobic organisms may have been wiped out by the appearance of oxygen. Around 1300 million years back, oxygen levels in the atmosphere reached 1%.

Recent studies suggest that interplay between biology and geology let the oxygen concentrations fluctuate periodically over the past 2 billion years. It commences with some oxygen in earth's atmosphere which reacted in the geosphere. Oxygen has a peculiar reactivity. It vividly reacts with iron in rocks or with hydrogen spewed out of volcanoes. When the earth calmed down, less geological oxygen reactions occurred. The extra oxygen fueled biological life. The abundant growth of microbes created carbon-rich rocks onto the sea floor. Later the rocks formed dry land and reacted with the oxygen out of the atmosphere and oxygen levels decreased again.

More complex cells with nuclei (eukaryotes) began to evolve and multicellular organisms emerged. The ozone (O_3) layer in the atmosphere formed and subsequently screened out much of the UV light and facilitated the emergence of life forms from the sea. Then 65 million years ago primates appeared and only 5 million years ago humans came on the scene. At that time the atmospheric oxygen concentration was 20.8%. During evolution oxygen slowly increased in the atmosphere and living organisms could gradually adapt to the apparent toxic properties of oxygen.

The unusual reactivity of oxygen necessitates its continuous formation by photosynthesis. At the same time we use its reactivity in various physiological processes. Oxygen is reduced by four electrons in a stepwise fashion (Fig. 2.1).

Oxygen has two unpaired electrons. This explains the ease by which oxygen can readily take up additional electrons. Oxygen with one additional electron is called superoxide radical. Oxygen with two electrons is called the peroxide anion; this form can lead to the formation of hydrogen peroxide.

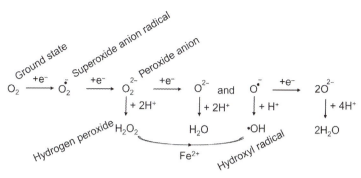

FIGURE 2.1   Scheme of stepwise reduction of O_2. In this scheme the formation of superoxide anion radicals, peroxide anions, hydrogen peroxide, and water is illustrated.

With three electrons the very reactive hydroxyl radical is generated. And finally, with four electrons oxygen is transformed into water.

So-called transition metals like iron or copper can activate the formation of reactive oxygen species (ROS). Luckily in our body the iron is generally safely stored away in proteins limiting the reactivity of the transition metal. Energy (light) may also activate oxygen, generating the so-called singlet oxygen forms.

All these reactive oxygen forms are called "ROS." In the lay press these forms are regularly indicated as oxygen radicals. This is not correct because not all of these intermediate oxygen species contain a free unpaired electron, which is the definition of a radical. They are reactive though, some more than others.

Because of its facile reaction with electrons, oxygen can be used as an electron sink in physiological processes. This is applied in mitochondria, cellular organelles which are crucial for energy, in the form of ATP production. Mitochondria are the power houses of the cell. The electron transport chain in the mitochondria is the driving force for mitochondrial ATP synthesis. The flow of electrons, through this chain, eventually goes to oxygen which is thereby transformed into water. Partial reduction of oxygen in this process may lead to ROS and may lead to damage.

Oxygen binds to iron. As mentioned, this already played a role in regulating the oxygen in the development of the earth's oxygen atmosphere. Also in the transport of oxygen in the body binding to iron plays a role. Iron is an intricate part of the protein hemoglobin which is the transporter for oxygen in red blood cells from lungs to the mitochondria. Heme (as part of hemoglobin) is a specific molecular structure that holds iron and allows iron to bind oxygen.

Another evolutionary old enzyme is the liver heme-containing protein cytochrome P450. The enzyme plays an important role in the liver (Chapter 3: The Coping Body—A Myriad of Exposures). It metabolizes both endogenous compounds like hormones or fatty acids as well as xenobiotics (compounds which are strange to the body like drugs or exogenous toxins). It is however also found in other organs. Moreover, the enzyme can be found over the entire phylogenetic scale: mammals, plants, and bacteria. The widespread availability suggests its early presence in evolution. This has recently been corroborated by genomics informatics. Its early role could have been that it offered protection against the toxicity of oxygen in favor of the anaerobic organisms. Interestingly, under strict anaerobic conditions this mammalian cytochrome P450 enzyme displays a different function which indeed is suggestive for this other evolutionary role for this old enzyme.

Oxygen has also gained a pivotal role in immune defense. Upon stimulation immune cells can produce various ROS. They form the last line of defense against invading microorganisms. The microorganisms are taken up by these cells like macrophages and bombarded with these oxidizing species

(A)

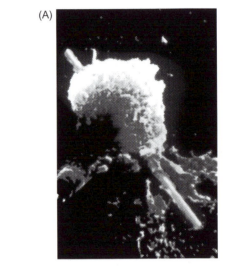

(B)

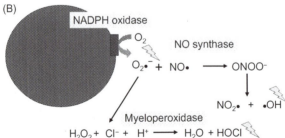

FIGURE 2.2   (**A**) Picture of macrophage trying to destroy asbestos particle. http://www.alamy. com/stock-photo-asbestos-49168810.html. (**B**) Illustration of various oxidizing species formed by phagocytic cells. *(A) From BSIP SA/Alamy Stock Photo.*

and destroyed. People who do not have this capability because they miss the enzyme producing these ROS in the immune cells cannot defend themselves properly and will die at an early age. This genetic disease is called chronic granulomatous disease. Sometimes macrophages can engulf a particle but cannot destroy it. This is the case with some asbestos fibers. The cells begin to produce the oxidizing species but the only result is that the surrounding tissue is affected by them (Fig. 2.2).

THE TOXICITY OF OXYGEN

The health risk of a compound is determined by its hazard and by the exposure to the compound. This sounds quite logical. In order to be a risk, the compound should have some hazardous properties and you at least should be exposed to the substance. In lay press this is frequently forgotten. News items on the health risk of flame retardants in the computer or plasticizers in a rain coat are just examples out of many. This type of news that is brought to us seems rather worrying but if there is no exposure to the compounds there is no risk.

$$Risk = hazard \times exposure$$

It would put news items into perspective if this general rule would be taken into account more often.

But what about oxygen? Yes, the gas is hazardous because of the ROS that can be generated from it. On top of that the exposure is immense. A relative high concentration to which we are enduringly exposed 24/7. In fact most of us die as a consequence of oxygen toxicity!

The theory that aging is caused by ROS is already in vogue for quite some time. ROS cause wear and tear phenomena in cells. Proteins are damaged by oxidation, cross link, and lose their function. Oxidation breaks down fatty acids and the resulting products interact with proteins.

This process can be observed by fluorescence microscopy of senescent tissues. The light produced under the fluorescent microscope lead an old researcher sigh "the older you grow the more you glow." Also the DNA is damaged continuously in living cells. It has been estimated that DNA is oxidatively damaged a thousand times per cell per day. An extensive repair system as the DNA polymerases and ligases correct these defects. Enzymes like poly-ADPribose polymerase (PARP) are employed by the cell to loosen the DNA enabling the repair machinery to function.

PARP is dependent for its function on ATP. Extensive DNA repair consumes intracellular ATP. Not only damage to nuclear DNA but also to mitochondrial DNA affects the genetic integrity. One of the consequences is that the risk for cancer increases with age. At the end of the maximal life span of various species (including humans) there is a cumulative risk of cancer of 30%. Interestingly the higher the basal metabolism (and thus more formation of ROS) of an organism (used calories per kg body weight per day) the lower the maximal life span.

Aging is a complex process and other explanations have also been brought to the fore like various programming theories, like sequential switching on and off of genes or hormonal control of aging or the programmed decline of the immune system. Even in these theories, ROS are involved. Overall, the paradox of aerobic life is that we need oxygen and die as a result of oxygen exposure (Fig. 2.3).

ROS are necessary for normal physiological functions. Their toxicity is restrained by the so-called antioxidants, compounds that prevent the oxidation of other compounds. A good example is butter. Oxygen will make the butter rancid. The polyunsaturated fatty acids in the butter oxidize. Light and heat augment the oxidation process. The butter is therefore kept in the refrigerator. Antioxidants are also added to the butter to protect it from deterioration. Vitamin E (also called alfa-tocopherol) is a fat-soluble antioxidant vitamin and inhibits the oxidation process. Also in our membranes, which consist of fatty acids, vitamin E inhibits the same oxidative damage.

Other antioxidants are vitamin C (ascorbic acid), beta-carotene, and so-called polyphenols. These compounds are abundantly found in fruits and vegetables. The antioxidants work in conjunction and form a network that protects against oxidation.

We are also equipped with an intricate system of antioxidant enzymes, which are, not surprisingly, evolutionary early proteins. Aerobic metabolism is regarded as a system that should be in balance. Oxygen and oxygen-derived reactive species are at the same time a necessity and a danger. In the 1985 the term "oxidative stress" was coined in a book by H. Sies. This expression "oxidative stress" was defined as a disturbance in oxidant—antioxidant balance in favor of the former. It gives rise to the feeling that the stress (which has a negative connotation) should be resisted. The strategy seems simple: antioxidants should do the job. And the marketing for antioxidants is easy: oxidative stress

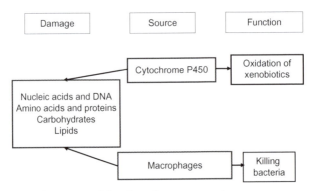

FIGURE 2.3   Function versus toxicity of reactive oxygen species.

is bad, antioxidants protect against oxidative stress, take antioxidants, and health effects are guaranteed.

It could have been anticipated that it is not that simple because it was known already at that time that normal physiology also needs oxidants. However, oxidative stress has been associated with many chronic, frequently age-related, diseases.

Quite a few chemicals are toxic via the formation of ROS in a process called "redox cycling." Compounds first take up an electron and shuttle this to oxygen, whereby oxygen becomes activated. In this way the toxicity of the herbicide paraquat is explained. Paraquat is banned in Europe but still heavily used in Brazil. Human exposure leads to lung toxicity via this mechanism. Adequate treatment is cumbersome.

The cardiotoxicity of the antitumor drug doxorubicin (Chapter 1: From Pretaster to Toxicologist) also occurs via this process of redox cycling. The process is dose limiting on the use of doxorubicin and forms one of the major drawbacks of this effective cytostatic.

The antibiotic nitrofurantoin, frequently used in the treatment of urinary tract infections, can display toxic side effects, for example in the lungs, via redox cycling. The same process has been described for cocaine. In some cases, where the endogenous antioxidant protection is substandard, nitrofurantoin, or cocaine toxicity may be brought to the fore.

ADAPTATION PROCESSES

Not only in science but also in marketing the term "ROS" is used quite frequently. As shown in Fig. 2.1 these species in fact differ and their chemical properties are very diverse. The more detailed knowledge is obtained on the subject, the more differentiation between all these forms of oxygen is required.

Questions as to their source, their reactivity toward all kind of biomolecules, and their interaction with antioxidants are all of biological importance. As a matter of fact, the terminology "antioxidants" is much too broad. Each antioxidant has its own reactivity. This might be an important factor in understanding their action.

People use antioxidants in general but in fact every compound with an antioxidant profile has its own characteristic. Also, the use of antioxidants should be refined. An interesting example in this respect is the use of vitamin E in persons that experienced an ischemic heart disease in two groups, a British and an Italian high-risk patient population. The British group (Cambridge to be precise) profited more than the Italian group of the supplementation. It was explained that unlike the British group the Italian population already had the benefit of an antioxidant-rich Mediterranean diet, and additional supplementation was less effective. A form of what we would call personalized nutrition.

As said, the extensive use of the term "oxidative stress" set in motion a certain type of research that was directed to counteract the stress. We now realize that in cells several oxidation and reduction processes play a role. So-called redox processes and not only oxidation. The redox processes regulate all kinds of cellular reactions.

In fact, gene regulation and thereby protein modulation is steered by redox processes. Several cellular "master switches" that regulate gene expression are under redox control. These master switches are NF-κB and Nrf2. Oxidative damage activates these switches. NF-κB activation leads to inflammation and activation of Nrf2 tunes-up gene expression leading to endogenous antioxidant enzymes. In this way adaptation to oxidative damage occurs (Fig. 2.4).

Oxidative stress and inflammation are intricately coupled. Oxidative stress leads to inflammation (via NF-κB) and activation of inflammatory cells cause oxidative stress. Table 2.1 presenting diseases associated with oxidative stress might also be read as illnesses associated with inflammation.

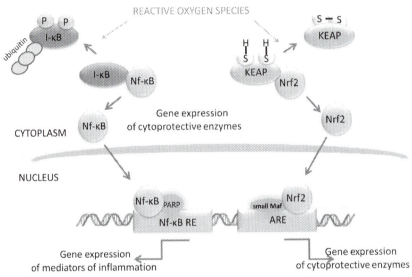

FIGURE 2.4 Figure explaining the activation of the transcription factors by oxidative stress and their cellular consequences.

TABLE 2.1 Examples of oxidative stress associated diseases

Several disorders in the lungs and the cardiovascular system associated with oxidative stress

- Lung: COPD, idiopathic pulmonary fibrosis, bronchopulmonary dysplasia, inhaled oxidants (like ozone), cigarette smoke, chemicals (e.g., paraquat and bleomycin), and adult respiratory distress syndrome, sarcoidosis
- Cardiovascular system: Myocardial infarction, atherosclerosis, (pre-)eclampsia, and chemicals (doxorubicin)

Mild damage of the Nrf2 system gives activation of this gene expression system and upregulates the endogenous antioxidant system. In other words a mild oxygen stress (not enough to kill a cell of course) enhances protective mechanism. In the redox field this is now widely accepted. This process is called eustress (good stress) or hormesis. From an evolutionary point of view this process of adaptation makes perfect sense. A continuous adaptation to oxygen took place in evolution. This process has of course an enormous impact on the way we perceive risks. A little oxygen toxicity might even be good for you.

Physical exercise also leads to oxidative stress. Increased energy demand during exercise activates mitochondrial activity which leads to ROS. Even a single bout of exercise has thus the capability to induce adaptation. This explains the training effect of mild exercise. Exhaustive exercise though might lead to damage. A delicate balance between adaptation and damage exists.

Discussion is ongoing whether antioxidants could be used to protect against the damage part without affecting the training result.

Many food-derived antioxidants like polyphenols are good activators of Nrf2. In fact polyphenols after being oxidized (that is after they have already acted as an antioxidant) activate Nrf2. In this way they further enhance the endogenous antioxidant system.

The paradox of aerobic life becomes even more intricate. We need oxygen to survive (the ATP synthesis relies on it), but at the same time oxygen offers an extreme health risk and indeed many diseases of aging have been related to oxygen toxicity (oxidative stress). Concurrent with a mild oxygen toxicity is the hormetic response, that is an induction of endogenous antioxidant systems.

The adventure in the oxygen bar definitely needs further scrutiny; which process prevails?

REFERENCES AND FURTHER READING

Bast, A., Haenen, G.R.M.M., 2013. Ten misconceptions about antioxidants. Trends Pharmacol. Sci. 34 (8).

Cabfield, D.E., Ngombi-Pemba, L., Hammerlund, E.U., Bengtson, S., Chaussidon, M., Gauthier-Lafaye, F., et al., 2013. Oxygen dynamics in the aftermath of the great oxidation of earth's atmosphere. Proc. Natl. Acad. Sci. U.S.A. 110 (42), 16736–16741.

Calabrese, E.J., 2015. Historic foundations of hormesis. Homeopathy 104 (2), 83–89.

Drent, M., Wijnen, P.A.H.M., Bast, A., 2012. Interstitial lung damage due to cocaine abuse: pathogenesis, pharmacogenomics and therapy. Curr. Med. Chem. 19 (33), 5607–5611.

Gotoh, O., 2012. Evolution of cytochrome P450 genes from the viewpoint of genome informatics. Biol. Pharm. Bull. 35 (6), 812–817.

Halliwell, B., 2000. The antioxidant paradox. Lancet 355 (9210), 1179–1180.

Halliwell, B., Gutteridge, J.M.C., 2015. Free Radicals in Biology and Medicine, fifth ed. Oxford University Press. Oxford, UK.

Jin, K., 2010. Modern biological theories of aging. Aging Dis. 1 (2), 72–74.

Lamprecht, M. (Ed.), 2015. Antioxidants in Sport Nutrition. CRC Press.

Rattan, S.I.S., Le Bourg, E. (Eds.), 2014. Hormesis in Health and Disease. CRC Press.

Sies, H., 2015. Oxidative stress: a concept in redox biology and medicine. Redox Biol. 4, 180–183.

Sies, H. (Ed.), 1985. Oxidative Stress. Academic Press, London.

Verissimo, G., Bast, A., Weseler, A.R., 2017. Paraquat disrupts the anti-inflammatory action of cortisol in human macrophages in vitro: therapeutic implications for paraquat intoxications. Tox. Res 6, 232–241.

Wickramashighe, R.H., Villee, C.A., 1975. Early role in evolution for cytochrome P450 in oxygen detoxification. Nature 256 (5517), 509–510.

<http://greatist.com/health/faq-whats-oxygen-bar> (last accessed June 14, 2016).

Chapter 3

The Coping Body—A Myriad of Exposures

A full-term healthy 13-day-old breast-fed baby died after his mother had been prescribed codeine (60 mg twice daily for 2 days and subsequently 30 mg twice daily) to treat episiotomy pain. The baby experienced feeding difficulties and lethargy at day 7 and was found dead on day 13. Analyses of the baby's blood (postmortem) and the mother's breast milk revealed toxic levels of morphine in both. Genetic testing of the mother showed that she was an ultra-rapid metabolizer of codeine.

This case report on the death of a neonate described in the medical journal *The Lancet* led to widespread concerns in obstetric and pediatric circles and scientific discussions up to the present time.

METABOLISM OF XENOBIOTICS

Ingestion is just one route of administration. Drugs are frequently administered conveniently via this oral route, indicated as per os (p.o.). Drugs can also be administered via an intraperitoneal, intramuscular, subcutaneous, and sublingual or intravenous (i.v.) injection (Fig. 3.1).

Toxins can enter the body similarly, for example, via a sting or a bite. More general exposure besides the p.o. route include contact via the skin (dermal exposure) or via inhalation (nose or lungs). In these types of exposures, protective barriers exist. The skin is slowly penetrable, but with soaps or fat-soluble compounds the penetration is enhanced. The air turbulence in the nose enhances particle impact and the nose cilia (small hairs) keep particles out. The inside of the lungs is covered with a small protective fluid layer that covers the inside cell layer of the lungs, the so-called epithelial cells. This protective covering fluid is called the epithelial lining fluid.

Via injection the various protective shields that exist to defend the body to xenobiotics are literally punctured and exposure is a fact. Intended use (of medication for instance) may employ injection to ease uptake. Compounds that enter the body via ingestion and the gastrointestinal route (the enteral route) can be absorbed from the intestines into the bloodstream.

Intestinal absorption forms the port entry for nutrients. The large surface area of the intestines eases absorption of compounds. The blood (the

Toxicology: What Everyone Should Know. DOI: http://dx.doi.org/10.1016/B978-0-12-805348-5.00003-X

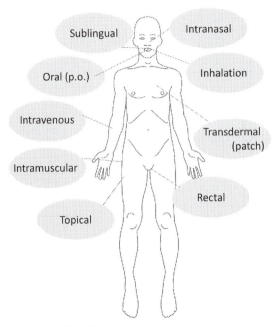

FIGURE 3.1 Routes of administration.

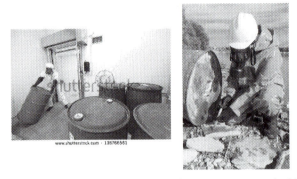

FIGURE 3.2 Man in protective clothing with gas mask—prevent exposure via skin and lungs.

portal vein) brings the absorbed compounds to the liver where further catabolism (breakdown of the compounds) or anabolism (synthesis of new compounds out of absorbed building blocks) occurs. Many of these reactions which are used to convert nutrients are also utilized to metabolize xenobiotics.

Following absorption the compound (Fig. 3.2) is distributed over the body. Thus toxic responses can take place in specific organs that function as

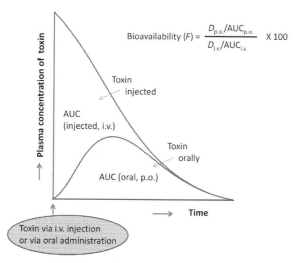

Bioavailability $(F) = \dfrac{D_{p.o.}/AUC_{p.o.}}{D_{i.v.}/AUC_{i.v.}} \times 100$

FIGURE 3.3 Schematic drawing of the plasma concentration time curve for i.v. and p.o. administration. AUC and F ($100 \times (D_{i.v.}/AUC_{i.v.})/(D_{p.o.}/AUCp.o.))$ are indicated.

vulnerable targets for specific compounds. The metal lead gives toxicity on the central nervous system; ethanol leads to liver toxicity; asbestos or ozone leads to lung toxicity; nickel may lead to skin toxicity; etc. The fate of compounds in the body is shortly designated as ADME. Absorption (A) and distribution (D) are discussed in conjunction with metabolism (M) and elimination (E).

Our body is equipped with an elaborate system to chemically convert fat-soluble compounds into more water-soluble compounds. This process of metabolism occurs primarily in the liver (hepatic metabolism). But other organs (e.g., intestine or lungs likewise) display metabolic activity as well. As mentioned, after ingestion a part of the dose will be absorbed and flows via the portal vein through the liver where it will be (partly) metabolized. The latter is called first-pass metabolism. The fraction of the dose that reaches the systemic circulation (with exception of the portal vein) is specified as the bioavailability of the compound.

Interestingly, with a rectal administration (via a suppository) it is possible to prevent this first-pass metabolism because the blood flow from the rectum does not directly go through the liver. This would be a nice way to administer medication but is clearly socially less acceptable (Fig. 3.3).

The process of metabolism or biotransformation alters xenobiotics into more water-soluble metabolites which will ease the elimination of compounds via the kidneys into the urine so that the fat-soluble compounds can leave the body via solution in water. Cytochrome P450 in the liver is an important enzyme catalyzing the biotransformation of xenobiotics toward a higher water solubility. The enzyme is found in membrane filaments, the endoplasmic reticulum, in the liver cell. The membrane constitutes a lipophilic environment enabling fat-soluble compounds to bind to cytochrome P450.

As discussed in Chapter 2, Death by Dose—The Most Toxic Compounds, the enzyme cytochrome P450 is an evolutionary ancient heme-containing protein. The iron (Fe) atom in the porphyrin structure (the heme moiety) forms the central place through which oxidation of xenobiotics can occur. The Fe atom is first reduced (in other words it becomes Fe^{2+}) and is then able to bind oxygen (O_2). The O_2 becomes activated on the Fe site to a reactive species which is used to oxidize a lipophilic xenobiotic, the substrate of the cytochrome P450 enzyme (RH). This metabolic reaction is usually designated as a phase 1 reaction. This oxidation can result in many types of functionalization reactions, by which the substrated is changed and more water-soluble reaction products (ROH) are formed. The compound NADPH is used to deliver electrons which are necessary for the reduction of Fe^{3+} and the activation of O_2.

The reaction is often described as:

$$RH + O_2 + NADPH + H^+ \rightarrow ROH + H_2O + NADP^+$$

RH symbolizes a wide variety of compounds that can thus be oxidized. Cytochrome P450 has been discovered in the liver in the mid-1950s by Axelrod and Brodie et al. The name of this important enzyme was derived from the finding that the pigment could bind carbon monoxide (CO) in its reduced Fe^{2+} form which showed an absorption maximum at a wavelength of 450 nm.

Cytochrome P450 is in fact not one enzyme but a whole family of isoenzymes. Small differences in the protein structure lead to variations in these enzymes. These iso-forms of cytochrome P450 have different substrate structure specificity, that is, they will metabolize diverse substrates and give various metabolites. These iso-cytochrome P450 forms are indicated with numbers and letters as CYP3A4, CYP2E1, or CYP2D6. The symbol CYP indicates the superfamily; the number indicates the gene family; a capital letter the subfamily; and the last numeral the individual gene.

The metabolite ROH can subsequently couple to other molecules like a glucuronic acid, a sulfate group, an acetate moiety, or a glutathione molecule. These coupling reactions are indicated as conjugation or phase 2 reactions (Fig. 3.4).

It has been established that animal species differ in their metabolic enzyme profile. Cats and lions can not catalyze glucuronidation; a pig hasn't the ability for sulfation; and dogs have no acetylation capacity. Not only phase 2 reactions differ between species, but also cytochrome P450 reactions (earlier classified as phase 1 reactions) diverge. Even within one species large variations in metabolism can occur.

A good example is CYP2D6, which is an important member of the cytochrome P450 enzyme superfamily. There is quite some variability in the

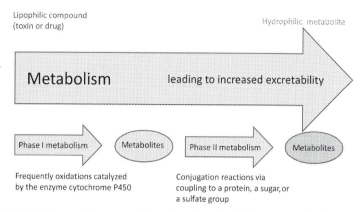

FIGURE 3.4   Scheme of phase 1 and phase 2 reactions in relation to water solubility.

efficiency and the amount of CYP2D6. This phenomenon is known as genetic polymorphism. Hence certain individuals will metabolize CYP2D6 substrates (xenobiotics that are metabolized by CYP2D6) quickly (ultra-rapid metabolizers) while others metabolize these substrates slowly (poor metabolizers). If the substrate is detoxified via CYP2D6 metabolism, the poor metabolizer may experience noxious effects. Ethnicity is feature in the occurrence of CYP2D6 variability. Approximately 8% of the Caucasians are poor metabolizers whereas this is 2% of the Asians.

Furthermore, substrates may also compete for the same enzyme thus inhibiting each other's metabolism. The activity of various CYP isoenzymes may also become increased via inducing the biosynthesis of an isoenzyme. This is called induction. This process can be regarded as a form of adaptation to a long-term exposure of a compound. The cytochrome P450 system becomes more active in an effort to metabolize the compound more efficiently. Likewise other substrates for the same isoenzyme will also be converted more rapidly.

RENAL ELIMINATION AND TREATMENT OF INTOXICATIONS

There are many ways by which compounds (or their metabolites) are eliminated or excreted by the body. Expel is possible via urine, tears, perspiration, saliva, respiration, milk, feces, or bile. The kidneys excrete compounds via glomerular filtration and by active tubular secretion. Filtration is only possible for compounds that are not bound to proteins in blood plasma, the so-called free fraction. Lipophilic uncharged molecules can passively be reabsorbed from the tubular fluid. The reason is that a large portion of the tubular fluid is also reabsorbed and consequently the concentration of the lipophilic substances increases and diffuses back (Fig. 3.5).

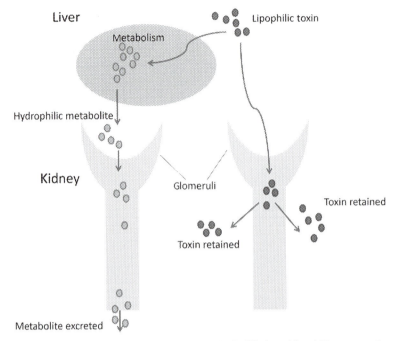

FIGURE 3.5   Schematic on the renal excretion and back diffusion of lipophilic compounds.

Weak acids are excreted when the tubular fluid becomes too alkaline because this leads to ionization of the acid and reduces passive reabsorption. The ionized (charged) molecule cannot pass through the membrane back into the blood stream and will be excreted into the urine. The opposite happens with weak bases. This effect is sometimes used to force excretion poisoning treatment. Urinary excretion of a weak acid can be forced by alkalizing the urine. Forced diuresis of a weakly basic drug is achieved by acidifying the urine.

This is an example of increasing the excretion to treat poisoning via pH. Two other fundamental treatments (viz. modifying ADME) of intoxications are reducing the absorption and the administration of antidotes. Absorption after ingestion of a toxic compound can be reduced by vomiting. This is only meaningful within 1 hour after ingestion. The vomiting reflex can be elicited by means of, for example, a spoon. After ingestion of petroleum products vomiting is dissuaded because of the risk of aspiration (i.e., inhaling of the fluid). Vomiting is also not advised after ingestion of corrosive compounds because of possible damage to the esophagus.

Activated charcoal (preferably administered in a health care facility) can also be used to decrease absorption. The charcoal binds the toxic compound and in that way reduces absorption. For children a dose of 1 g of activated charcoal per kg body weight with a maximum of 50 g is used. For adults the dose is 50 g of activated charcoal.

The use of antidotes is sometimes possible when the molecular mechanism of the toxicity is well known. This is frequently the case with drugs. Clinically the most occurring intoxication is with the pain killer paracetamol (acetaminophen). An overdose leads to irreversible liver injury. The mechanism of toxicity is well described. In the liver, paracetamol is metabolized to a reactive metabolite that reacts with sulfur groups of proteins in the liver. This leads to liver damage (hepatotoxicity). By abundantly supplying sulfur groups via an i.v. infusion with *N*-acetylcysteine it is anticipated that the hepatic sulfur groups will be restored and the eventual fatal toxicity can be reversed.

An interesting example is the toxicity of excess of bilirubin in the blood (bilirubinemia). This can occur in the new born. Normally bilirubin, the destruction product the hemoglobin of erythrocytes, is conjugated to glucuronic acid in the liver and thus excreted in the bile. In the new born this conjugation (a phase 2 reaction) is not fully developed yet. It has been suggested that a slightly higher concentration of bilirubin might be beneficial because it protects against oxygen damage that occurs during birth (from a low oxygen environment in passage of the birth channel to open air). Too much bilirubin however may be toxic and can lead to neuronal damage. In early days the glucuronidation reaction was induced by administration of a barbiturate, a sleeping drug.

PREDICTION OF METABOLISM AND TOXICITY— DO WE NEED ANIMAL TESTING?

It is obvious that differences in the absorption, distribution, metabolism, and elimination of compounds between species hamper use of laboratory animals for prediction of ADME in humans. Moreover, the variability in metabolism necessitates an individual approach to determine the biotransformation of a compound. This personalized approach is increasingly used to tailor the optimal dose of pharmaceutics. Undoubtedly, in the (foreseeable) future the genetic profiling of metabolic enzymes for everyone will be available. This will enable physicians and pharmacists to suggest a safe and effective dose of a pharmaceutical compound. In addition the phenotypical variation (induction or inhibition by dietary factors or other drugs) will also be categorized on an individual basis, which will further fine tune the pharmacotherapy.

For unintentional exposure to compounds clearly larger safety margins have to be used to extrapolate animal data to the human situation or to generalize safe human exposures (Chapter 5: From Prevention to Precaution— Valuing Risks).

Knowledge on metabolism is pivotal but still just one aspect of understanding how compounds may affect human health. We currently mainly rely on traditional animal testing for toxicological evaluation of compounds. In most countries the three Rs form an explicit managing principle in the use of animals in science: Replacement, Reduction, and Refinement. When we translate that to toxicology, the three Rs read as follows.

Replacement: Avoid or replace the use of animals in toxicological research.

There is a keen worldwide interest to develop methods for toxicity assessments with quick and efficient tests. Interesting developments are "organs-on-chips," human cells grown in such a way that the system mimics structure and function of human organs and organ systems to test compounds.

Furthermore, computer models have been developed that simulate human biology to predict how compounds react in the human body. In the meantime impressive databases on prediction of metabolic routes of compounds have been developed. To illustrate the function: In the program, a molecular structure of a random molecule is drawn and the program predicts the likelihood of the formation of certain metabolites.

In addition, quantitative structure−activity relationships are computer estimations of the probability for a compound to be hazardous. This requires chemical knowledge in conjunction with availability of extensive databases with data on exiting substances. These databases are currently packed in various large research programs in Europe and in the United States.

In the United States this is among others performed in the Tox21 program, a federal collaboration among the US Environmental Protection Agency, National Institutes of Health, including National Center for Advancing Translational Sciences and the National Toxicology Program at the National Institute of Environmental Health Sciences, and the US Food and Drug Administration. One of the aims of this program is to screen approximately a 10,000 compound library against 30 cell-based assays. Many cellular responses for all these substances are determined in what is called a quantitative high- throughput screening format. In this way structure−activity signatures are obtained that could act as predictive surrogates for in vivo (in animal) toxicity.

New analytical techniques make it possible to measure very low concentrations of compounds and enable the use of "microdosing." A minute dose of a substance is administered to a human volunteer and will provide information on metabolite formation, speed of elimination, and safety. A major drawback is that low-dose responses might differ from high-dose effects (Chapter 6, Molecular Trepidations—The Linear Nonthreshold Model).

Reduction: Use methods by which we can obtain comparable toxicological information from fewer animals or more information from the same number of animals.

Things that come to mind are to avoid unnecessary replications of experiments although common scientifically statistical methods dictate this. Use a good experimental design and planning. Fortunately, animal ethical committees look over the shoulder of the individual experimenter to improve the latter further. New techniques also lead to reduction like modern imaging or telemetry. In the latter case telemetry devices are implanted in the animal that enable continuous monitoring of various parameters as temperature, movement, blood pressure, electrocardiogram, oxygen pressure, and so forth. With these, still costly techniques, a lot of information can be obtained from one animal and the animal serves as its own control thus reducing the necessity to have a control group. In toxicology this technique is very helpful because many parameters are sampled simultaneously. This is excellently suited for this type of research because it is not known on forehand how and when a specific toxic response show up.

Refinement: Use methods in which potential pain, suffering, or distress is minimized for the toxicological studies in animals, and enhance animal welfare.

There is societal criticism on the three Rs stating that the 3Rs principles focus on the humane use of animals and do not aptly address the ethics of using animals as such. By animal researchers reduction is frequently interpreted as reduction of the numbers of animals used per study while by others it is understood as an absolute reduction in the number of animals used.

A rising communal awareness of inhumane practices and concern for animal welfare is apparent, although this awareness is far from new. In a time when criticism against animal testing (vivisection) was not really considered seriously (the 19th and the first half of the 20th century), the famous Lewis Carroll (*Alice in Wonderland*; *Through the Looking Glass*) brought to bear quite a few analytical arguments against the use of animals in research that still ring true today, albeit some of them contrary to, for instance, the animal rights movement.

Stephen M. Wise and his organization the Nonhuman Rights Project who persuaded a New York judge to promulgate a historic ruling tentatively suggesting that a confined chimpanzee named Tommy might possess the basic common law right of habeas corpus. A legal status for nonhuman animals on fundamental rights as bodily integrity and bodily liberty will fundamentally change our perspective on the use of animals in toxicology. To be sure, rights conferred to animals, such as bodily integrity and bodily liberty, open the door to ad absurdum arguments such as Carroll, not tongue-in-cheek, proposes as not being allowed to "light a candle in a summer evening for mere pleasure, lest some hapless moth should rush to an untimely end!" The solution would be, illogically in Carroll's view, to "assign rights to animals in proportion to their size."

Nevertheless, moving away from the utilitarian age of animal testing seems the way forward in our work on toxicology. Unfortunately, considering many legal standards and societal demands on safety, some testing in animals will need to continue in the foreseeable future, as it is presently not possible to adequately describe how compounds are metabolized in the body using alternatives.

THE CASE REPORT

Can we now explain the case report as presented in the beginning of this chapter? Mother receives codeine. This drug is metabolized by CYP2D6 into morphine. Because the mother is an extensive metabolizer the levels of morphine out of codeine will be high. Morphine can be excreted into the breast milk which is administered to the neonate. Normally morphine undergoes a glucuronidation (a phase 2 reaction). Neonates might possess a not fully functional glucuronidation and the morphine levels might remain too high in the newborn which might have been the cause of death: a morphine overdose. An interesting detail is that two morphine glucuronides can be formed, morphine-3-glucuronide and morphine-6-glucuronide. The latter still has morphine-like activities. This is exceptional because most glucuronides do not have the activity of the parent compound anymore. The glucuronides are excreted via the kidneys. Renal failure may lead to accumulation of the glucuronides.

Could we have predicted this fatal accident? Determination of CYP2D6 might at least have been a premonition.

REFERENCES AND FURTHER READING

Axelrod, J., 1955. The enzymatic demethylation of ephedrine. J. Pharmacol. 114, 430–438.

Bast, A., 1980. Is formation of reactive oxygen by cytochrome P450 perilous and predictable? Trends Pharmacol. Sci. 7, 266–270.

Bast, A., Haenen, G.R.M.M., Bruynzeel, A.M.E., van der Vijgh, W.J.F., 2007. Protection by flavonoids against anthracycline cardiotoxicity: from chemistry to clinical trials. Cardiovasc. Toxicol. 7 (2), 154–159.

Brodie, B., Axelrod, J., Cooper, J.R., Gaudette, L., LaDu, B.N., Mitoma, C., et al., 1955. Detoxication of drugs and other foreign compounds by liver microsomes. Science 121, 603–604.

Green R.L. (Ed.), 1965. Some popular fallacies about vivisection. In: The Works of Lewis Carroll. Spring books, London, pp. 1092–1100.

Huang, R., Xia, M., Sakamura, S., Zhao, J., Shahane, S.A., Attene-Ramos, M., et al., 2016. Modelling the Tox21 10K chemical profiles for in vivo toxicity prediction and mechanism characterization. Nat. Commun. 7, 10425.

Koren, G., Cairns, J., Chitayat, G., Leeder, S.J., 2006. Pharmacogenetics of morphine poisoning in a breast fed neonate of a codeine-prescribed mother. Lancet 368, 704.

Wijnen, P.A.H.M., Op den Buijs, R.A.M., Drent, M., Kuipers, P.M.J.C., Neefs, C., Bast, A., et al., 2007. Review article: The prevalence and clinical relevance of cytochrome P450 polymorphisms. Aliment. Pharmacol. Ther. 26 (Suppl. 2), 211–219.

⟨http://www.nonhumanrightsproject.org/⟩ (accessed July 24, 2016).

Chapter 4

Nature Knows Best—Chemicals From the Geobiological Sphere

The Harris family is out on their weekly shopping duties. Apart from the regular groceries, sodas, and toiletries they also shop for some luxury goods: some perfume for both the ladies and men in the household, a few bottles of wine, and a nice bouquet of flowers to liven up the dining room. Interestingly, their choices of these luxury products are determined to a major extent by chemistry. The "aroma" of wine, the "fragrance" of the perfumes of choice, and the "bouquet" of flowers are in fact none other than words that designate the pleasantries of certain chemicals (organic molecules) coming off these luxuries. The chemicals we sense with our nose have found their way into our everyday language. Concerning the wine, taste follows smell, and merge once the first sip is taken. The complex of no less than 25,000 chemicals determines whether we are dealing with a good wine.

But the Harris's are not done yet. They also frequent a specialty store that sells health products. There, they buy a few bottles of bioflavonoid capsules, antioxidants that purportedly improve cardiovascular health, and some bio-vitamin C, which they think is obviously better than the synthetic counterpart. Fortunately, the store also sells painkillers, so a bottle of aspirins is added to the purchases (Fig. 4.1).

In this chapter, we will take a close look at the chemical content of the produce the Harris's have bought. Despite the fact that chemistry is a highly specialized field of research, everyday terms we pointed at here represent the intimate relationship between man and his chemical environment: from the food we eat to the air we breathe, from dietary supplements to medicinal drugs we consume to improve health or cure a disease.

Interestingly, for decades now modern man divides the chemical sphere he lives in into two parts: the natural—regarded as benign for the most part—and the synthetic—man-made chemicals that usually are thought to spell danger. Based on its origin, any chemical is considered to be easily recognized as either safe or dangerous. So, pesticides used during crop production, or antibiotics given to cows with an infection, or food additives such as food coloring and flavor enhancers are generally regarded as a threat to human health.

We will unfold this peculiar dichotomy and show that these two seemingly divided worlds—natural vs synthetic and safe vs dangerous—overlap

Toxicology: What Everyone Should Know. DOI: http://dx.doi.org/10.1016/B978-0-12-805348-5.00004-1

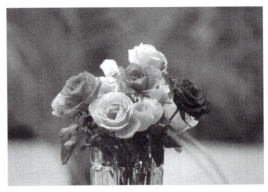

FIGURE 4.1 Pictures of bouquet of flowers and a bottle of quercetin (a flavonol).

far more than generally realized. Ironically, with the advent of the chemical industry and research in the 19th century, the discovery and production of an increasing number of different chemicals facilitated the growing realization that the natural world itself harbors an immense amount and diversity of chemicals. And this realization fed the growing field of toxicology throughout the 20th and 21st centuries. We will review both ends of the scale of the environment, i.e., the personal level on the one hand—food and drugs—and the global level on the other—the geobiological sphere.

THE CHEMICAL WORLD OF FOOD AND COFFEE

The way humans are exposed to the wealth of chemicals is mostly through the diet that varies widely across countries and continents. Just to give an idea of how much food is consumed: an individual eats, during his or her lifetime on average, some 30 tons of food.

The interest in food and its health impacts is a never-ending source for TV shows, glossy's, cookbooks, professional and academic articles. Man seems to have returned to the ancient idea that food is far more than needed for survival: food is life and should increase vitality and health for as long as possible. However, the fact that chemistry is addressed in all this is hardly ever mentioned. Indeed, humans have become very wary of everything chemical. Foods that have been "tainted" with pesticides, antibiotics, coloring and flavoring, and other processing techniques immediately raise our suspicions. The "natural" has been "polluted" with "the chemical." And that idea foolishly has become the mental furniture of our day and age.

Overall, most people will enthusiastically embrace the idea that the foods we buy at the store should be, and in fact usually are, quite safe. The food industry, governments, and consumer organizations advertise this widely. Yet, food is a complicated mix of many thousands of different chemicals with all sorts of biological activities, not easily categorized as either good or bad. Thus, apart from the nutrition we require daily, many other chemicals slip in our "system" that have all sorts of effects on our health, for better or for worse. This we have addressed to some extent in the first chapter. And we haven't even started cooking yet!

Indeed, preparing a meal in the kitchen or food being processed industrially—frying, baking, boiling, roasting—changes the chemical composition of our food quite extensively and increases the number of chemicals we consume. This fact alone brings us in a world beyond unprocessed foods as can be obtained at the supermarket or from local farmers.

The chemical changes in foods caused by moderate heat modify or intensify flavor chemicals that are natural to a food. The so-called browning reactions at higher temperatures produce new flavors that are characteristics of the cooking process. Caramelization is one example of a browning reaction. When we heat plain table sugar, sucrose, it first melts into a thick, colorless syrup. After a while it slowly changes color, becoming light yellow, and gradually intensifies to dark brown. At the same time, its flavor develops a full aroma with some acidity and a hint of bitterness. If this browning reaction goes too far, it produces an unpleasant bitter mixture. If kept in check, the complex chemistry renders a sugar-derived product applied in all sorts of candy and other sweets (Fig. 4.2).

Thus, with some cooking skills tasty results can be created. A cook is none other than a chemist producing many hundreds of chemicals in one go. And not all these newly formed chemicals add flavor and aroma to our dish. Let's look at one of the most common morning brews in the world: coffee.

It is valued for its uplifting and stimulating qualities and its specific flavor and aroma. The chemical responsible for the stimulating effect is caffeine and is a repellent to discourage pests and herbivores to eat that plant. But before we can actually prepare a good breakfast brew, a lot of processing of the coffee beans needs to be done.

Coffee beans are picked, processed, and dried once the berries of the *Coffea* plant that contain them are ripe. Dried coffee beans are roasted to varying

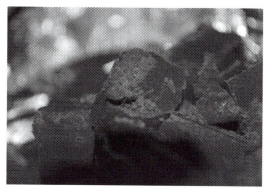

FIGURE 4.2 Picture of fudge.

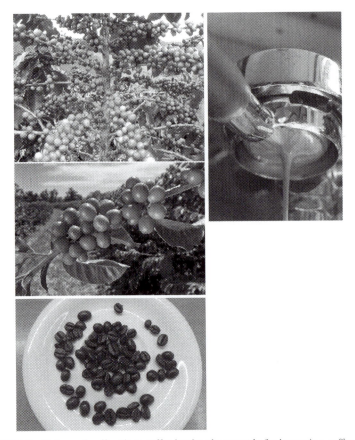

FIGURE 4.3   Pictures of coffee plant, coffee berries almost ready for harvesting, coffee beans, and an espresso shot from an E61 brew head.

degrees, depending on the desired flavor. It is only through roasting that the beans gain the characteristic and cherished aroma and flavor. Roughly a thousand chemical compounds have been identified within the roasted coffee bean that adds to the overall brew. And more are discovered every day (Fig. 4.3).

Within this overall mix, some chemicals formed during roasting have less than desirable characteristics. Polycyclic aromatic hydrocarbons (PAHs) for instance are formed during especially higher temperatures. PAHs are a group of carcinogenic organic compounds. It is estimated that intake of PAHs through the consumption of coffee is some 150 ng per day, i.e., 150 billionths of a gram. The total daily PAHs intake from all sources is estimated to be roughly 1700 ng, or 1.7 µg.

How dangerous these compounds in fact are, and how to assess those risks, is subject of Chapter 5, From Prevention to Precaution—Valuing Risks. What is known from research is that regular enjoyment of coffee does not increase

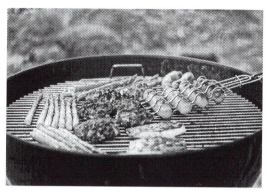

FIGURE 4.4   Picture of barbeque.

the rate of cancer. In fact, coffee consumption has all sorts of beneficial effects and that is good news for all of us who need their daily dose of java.

With our food processing both at home and in the factory, we chemically change our food. That, of course, is nothing new. With the discovery of fire, our ways to prepare food transformed and opened up new venues of flavors and aromas. However, the moment science turned its gaze on food and food processing, it revealed a far bigger chemical landscape than anticipated: the geobiological sphere.

Let's go back to coffee. The PAHs that can arise from roasting the beans are also found on barbequed meat. Cooking over a smoky wood fire deposits PAHs from the burning wood onto the meat. We could prevent this by cooking meat over a smokeless charcoal fire. But, if fat drips on the coals and burns, that will create PAHs that again will deposit on the meat. Or, PAHs are formed if the fat ignites on the meat surface itself.

So, barbequing requires quite a bit skill as to prevent unwanted chemicals. However, it also shows that the environment delivers quite a bit of chemistry to the dinner table not linked to the skills of the cook (Fig. 4.4).

An interesting example of this "environmental chemistry" involves organohalogens. These organic chemical compounds contain the elements fluorine, chlorine, bromine or iodine, the halogens. Focusing on the most abundant of the halogens, chlorine, it obtained its infamy in World War I when German troops used it in its elemental gaseous form as a chemical weapon on April 22, 1915, near Ypres against Allied troops.

In most households, chlorine is found in the form of bleach, the unmistakable smell of which we associate with a freshly cleaned restroom and, happily, not with war. Most cooks, either professional or amateur, also use chlorine in the form of sodium chloride, table salt, as to add flavor to the dish.

We need salt in order to stay healthy, and it is used in many different processes in our bodies. For instance, chloride is used in the stomach for the formation of hydrochloric acid. On average, we carry between 100 and 200 g of salt in our bodies depending on our mass.

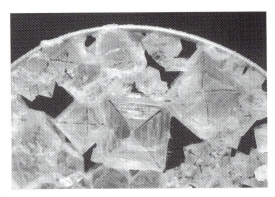

FIGURE 4.5 Picture of table salt crystals.

The chlorination of drinking water as to keep it free from water-borne diseases, such as typhoid, cholera, and meningitis, has been a common, cheap, and highly effective practice for almost a century. It does affect taste, but keeping infectious organisms away from drinking water is top priority in any country (Fig. 4.5).

The amount of salt in the world is staggering. Chloride in seawater amounts to some 1.8%. The world production of salt is close to 300,000,000 tons per year. It seems strange therefore that chlorinated hydrocarbons are thought to result from the chemical industry only. So, any organochlorides found in the environment must be the result of industrial pollution or the result of chlorination of drinking water, so the story goes.

One of the most notorious organochlorides is perhaps DDT (dichlorodi-phenyltrichloroethane in full), a now banned insecticide. Dioxin is another example that is regarded by some as the most toxic man-made chemical ever (more on that later). In the late 20th century a ban on production and use of all chlorinated hydrocarbons was strongly advocated by especially environmental NGOs.

However, once we penetrate deeper into the geobiological sphere, the more we come to understand that nature itself delivers an overwhelming amount of organochlorides from all kinds of sources: plants, molds, sea creatures, erupting volcanoes, forest fires, and so on. Some of these compounds are produced in amounts that dwarf human production such as chloro-methane. Indeed, it is estimated that some 75% of all chlorinated substances found in the environment come from biological sources and geological sources such as volcanic eruptions. And that includes dioxins. Many natural sources have been discovered that produce dioxins. It is even suggested that our own immune response is responsible for the generation of minute amounts!

Seafood is especially interesting as the marine environment contains so much chloride and the other halogens to a lesser extent. In other words, sea

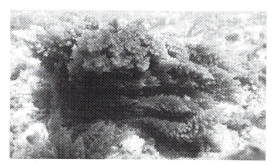

FIGURE 4.6 Picture of Limu kohu.

creatures and plants are literally surrounded by halogens. It is therefore no real surprise then that many different organohalogens have been discovered in edible seafood. For instance, the chemically prolific red algae *Asparagopsis taxiformis* and *Asparagopsis armata* ("Limu kohu"—pleasing seaweed), which are prized by Hawaiians for their flavor and aroma, contain the relatively novel (*E*)-1,2-dibromoethene, (*Z*)-1,2-dibromoethene, and tribromoethene.

Even more interestingly, a study confirmed one of the most heavily brominated enol esters (pentabromo-2-propenyl di- and tribromoacetate) ever found in nature produced by *A. taxiformis*. These two compounds were confirmed by chemical synthesis in the laboratory (Fig. 4.6).

Polybrominated biphenyl ethers (PBDEs) used as fire retardants have been restricted from commercial use by cause of their toxicity and bioaccumulation in the environment. However, PBDEs that mirror and even surpass the toxicity of man-made counterparts have been found naturally produced by marine sponges, especially of the order Dysideidae. Naturally produced PBDEs permeate the marine environment and even bioaccumulate in marine animals and are carried over to the human food chain. Recently, the genetic background of the natural synthesis of PBDEs has been mapped.

Should we worry then about this immense smorgasbord of chemicals that make up our food? We have been taught to fear "chemistry" and our food is teeming with all sorts of chemicals that, in some cases, include chloride, and we are not just talking about table salt. These chemicals are either innately present in the consumables, are delivered by environmental sources, or are added during the process of cooking.

Some decades ago, humans weren't aware of organohalogens at all. It was easy to focus on dioxins and DDT and a few other chemicals and try to ban them from our world by law, so we thought. Food was "clean" if it was produced naturally (organic, biological) and wasn't industrially processed. Our world was orderly divided between natural and synthetic, good and bad, healthy and unhealthy, clean and dirty.

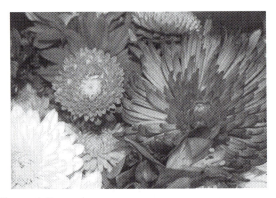

FIGURE 4.7   Picture of *Chrysanthemum.*

And humans still cling to this idea. People like to protect themselves by choosing those products that are portrayed as natural and as a result, it is thought, free from harm. Organic farming, despite of its higher-priced produce, has become popular based exactly on the notion of naturalness and safety. Also, we like to buy not just vitamin C as supplement but preferably bio-vitamin C, although it is impossible to indicate any chemical difference between them. The Harris's, in other words, seem to buy into this story.

The reality that innate plant protection naturally comes from pesticides that are produced by plants or sealife themselves is far from new. In our romantic worldview of food and food production, we seem however to have lost the basics. The world of bacteria, molds, plants, and animals is one of assault and defense. And chemistry plays a big role therein.

The flowering plants of the genus *Chrysanthemum*, for instance, have been known for centuries to repel and kill insects. The responsible pyrethrins isolated in the beginning of the 20th century form the basis for the pyrethroids, manufactured chemicals that are very similar in structure to the pyrethrins, but are more toxic to insects and last longer in the environment than pyrethrins. So, nature formed the toolbox for chemists to improve upon insect control in crops (Fig. 4.7).

Comparing the consumption of natural and synthetic pesticides, humans roughly consume 1500 mg of natural pesticides and their breakdown products every day compared to approximately 0.09 mg of synthetic pesticide residues. It seems then that our fear of "the chemical" is misplaced but also gives a false sense of security.

SELECTIVE TOXICITY

As food contains so many natural "toxic" chemicals, couldn't food be used as medicine? The answer to that question is simply yes. A quote attributed to Hippocrates "Let food be thy medicine and medicine be thy food" holds today more than ever especially in view of our increasing knowledgebase. Toxicity and medicine are usually not seen as closely linked, let alone food and toxicity. Medicine should be safe, just as food, seems to be the general consensus.

In medicine we look for chemicals, drugs, that have a very specific effect on a disease state. Thus, we want as little side effects as possible: that is safety. However, the particular effect we prize in good medication is nothing other than selective toxicity against the disease we want to cure. Medication, thus, is *targeted toxicity*: the more focused the toxicity, the better the medication, and the fewer the side effects. These side effects are nothing other than broad and thereby undesirable toxicity.

Paul Ehrlich initiated this notion of targeted toxicity with his discovery of receptors at the beginning of the 20th century. It opened up a whole new world of understanding and disease treatment. To Ehrlich, receptors were small, chemically defined areas on large molecules (proteins). He wrote that "combining group of the protoplasmic molecule to which the introduced group (the molecules of medication; authors) is anchored will hereafter be termed receptor." This image of receptors in essence hasn't changed much but became more detailed for many different kinds of receptors. The action of drugs is characterized by a selective action on a specific target, a receptor or enzyme that is involved in curing a patient's disease.

This medicinal targeted toxicity results in measurable effects toward health, if all goes well. Usually drugs have a large easily quantifiable effect on a specific target (a receptor or enzyme) and the effects are usually seen over a relatively short period of time, days, weeks, and sometimes months. A rapid action is desired because diseases should ideally be cured as fast as possible for the patient's sake. If, however, medication needs to be taken over longer periods of time (e.g., asthma medication), side effects need to be at a minimum as to make this long-term medicinal exposure at all possible.

Food chemicals are different, and fortunately so. These chemicals usually do not have any drastic effects after consumption as medication does. Food constituents act on various targets and display multiple effects on our health. Unlike drugs, the actions of dietary components are mild. Looking at more detail, these effects can easily be categorized, surprisingly enough, as subtly toxic. It seems that we need to be pushed in order to stay healthy.

The health effect of food should also be tested differently compared to drug testing. The placebo-controlled double-blind randomized clinical trial (RCT) is commonly used for drugs, in which the effect of a drug is tested against a placebo without the patients and researchers knowing who gets what is not really appropriate for testing food and food constituents. The latter always are part of the diet and cannot easily be omitted for research reasons. You cannot leave out vitamins from the diet for example. Apart from the chemical complexity to actually do that, although not impossible, it would be unethical.

It is increasingly advocated that in order to investigate the effect of food, the organism is put under stress and various biomarkers that reflect the effect of the stressor are determined. The effect of food on the ability to withstand the stressor is subsequently measured. Examples of stressors are the administration a fatty, sugar containing, drink that elicits mild inflammation or smoking a few cigarettes or exhaustive exercise.

Another approach to evaluate the health effect of food is to quantify the effect on many of the physiological responses involved in a disease state. In this way a health index can be defined which takes into account multiple targets.

Doing sports (increasing our oxygen exposure) and eating well increases our endogenous protective system and thus renders protection in the long run against aging and disease.

So, the old definition of health of the WHO as a "state of complete physical, mental, and social well-being and not merely the absence of disease or infirmity" is wide off the mark. We do not live in a static world but in a dynamic one. And we behave accordingly by adapting to new situations the best we can. Health is thus *the ability to adapt*.

FOOD AND MEDICINE: THE "GOOD," THE "BAD," AND THE UNAVOIDABLE

Food is truly a complex mixture of chemicals that have all sorts of health effects. The longstanding golden rule is to diversify our daily diet and for good reasons: we hedge out bets. The wider the spread of consumed food chemicals, the smaller the chance we run afoul with health-impairing consumption habits.

A number of reasons carry this argument: (1) we reduce the chance to be exposed to the same food chemicals over and over again whereby (2) we reduce the chance of missing out on chemicals such as vitamins and minerals and antioxidants that are essential for our well-being, and (3) we reduce the chance of being exposed to chemicals we better do without such as potato alkaloids but also chemicals that are produced by molds such as the liver toxin aflatoxin.

Beneath these three arguments lies the notion that by diversifying our food intake, we train our bodies to deal with all sorts of chemicals. The potato alkaloids or the nasty courgette cucurbitacins or even the much feared mould aflatoxins can, at very small doses, trigger damage-repairing responses that in the end is beneficial for our health. As the maxim goes: what does not kill you makes you stronger.

Not that we should directly search out exposure to these compounds. That is not even required; we are exposed to such chemicals anyway. They are unavoidable. But it does show that "good" and "bad" chemicals as such do not exist: only the dose makes the poison. Even more so, traditionally classified bad chemicals actually can be a source for good for us, as long as the dosages are low enough. We have the ability to adapt, and this adaptability when trained enough will stimulate our health and longevity.

So the fear of "the chemical," our chemophobia is indeed a phobia, an anxiety disorder. We persistently fear "the chemical" in our food. This fear is narrowed down to pesticides sprayed during crop production, antibiotics used in animal rearing, food additives, and we will go to great lengths to avoid these chemicals, disproportional to the actual danger posed.

The disproportion is related to the fact that we have forgotten that food in all its naturalness carries with it all the chemistry we need to survive and thrive. From the carbohydrates, fats and protein to the vitamins and minerals and all the rest that might intoxicate us if we are not careful or might help us adapt to greater health. As human beings we are well adapted, within limits.

REFERENCES AND FURTHER READING

Agarwal V., Blanton J.M., Podell S., Taton A., Schorn M.A., Busch J., Lin Z., Schmidt E.W., Jensen P.R., Paul V., Biggs J.S., Golden J.W., Allen E.E., Moore B.S., Metagenomic discovery of polybrominated diphenyl ether biosynthesis by marine sponges, Nat Chem Biol. 13(5), 2017, 537–543.

Albert, A., 1981. Selective Toxicity. The Physico-chemical Basis of Therapy. Sixth ed. Chapman and Hall, London, New York.

Amsley, J., 2011. Nature's Building Blocks. Everything You Need to Know About the Elements. Oxford University Press, New York, NY.

Coffee. Emerging Health Effects and Disease Prevention. In: Chu, Y.-F. Institute of Food Technologists. Wiley-Blackwell, IFT Press, USA, Oxford, UK.

Dietz, B., Bolton, J.L., 2007. Botanical dietary supplements gone bad. Chem. Res. Toxicol. 20, 586–590.

Duke, J.A., Bogenschutz-Godwin, M.J., du Cellier, J., Duke, P.-A.K., 2003. CRC Handbook of Medicinal Spices. CRC Press, Boca Raton, FL, London, New York, Washington, DC.

Friedman, M., Mcdonald, G.M., Filadelfi-Keszi, M., 1997. Potato glycoalkaloids: chemistry, analysis, safety, and plant physiology. Crit. Rev. Plant Sci. 16 (1), 55–132.

Gribble, G.W., 2010. Naturally Occurring Organohalogen Compounds—A Comprehensive Update. SpringerWien, New York, NY.

Hanekamp, J.C., Bast, A., Calabrese, E.J., 2015. Nutrition and health—transforming research traditions. Crit. Rev. Food Sci. Nutr. 55 (8), 1074–1080.

European Food Safety Authority, 2008. Polycyclic aromatic hydrocarbons in food. Scientific Opinion of the Panel on Contaminants in the Food Chain. EFSA J. 724, 1–114.

Weseler, A.R., Bast, A., 2012. Pleiotropic-acting nutrients require integrative investigational approaches: the example of flavonoids. J. Agric. Food Chem 60 (36), 8941–8946.

Chapter 5

From Prevention to Precaution—Valuing Risks

The Nettles farm is home to some 100 dairy cows. The farmer and his family live a hard but fulfilling life, providing prime cheeses to the local market. Until one day the competent authorities pay the Nettles a visit on the suspicion of the use of illegal antibiotics. They take some urine samples and find parts per billion of some breakdown products (metabolites) of the drug furazolidone, which is not allowed in animal rearing. The reason for this ban is the suspicion of carcinogenic qualities of the primary drug and its metabolites. Therefore, in the European Union, a zero-tolerance policy is in place for chemicals such as this antibiotic. That simply means that the antibiotic and its metabolites should not be found in the cow's meat, organs, urine, and manure on any concentration level whatsoever, or as low as can be analyzed. As a result, the Nettles lost their cows—they were killed by order of government officials in order to protect public health—and almost their farm.

CHEMICALS—ASSESSING RISKS

The dose makes the poison. Probably the oldest and most famous discovery and axiom in toxicology stands at the heart of any analysis of risk when in contact with chemicals. Again, any chemical can be a risk to our health, even water. Thus, risk of chemicals in our environment—air, water, soil, food—is all about concentration levels of exposure. How do these different levels of exposure compare? How much for instance is a part per million (ppm), or billion (ppb), or trillion (ppt), the much-used terms in describing concentrations of all sorts of (un)wanted chemicals in our environment.

Let's start with a ppm (10^{-6}). In terms of the International System of Units, i.e., 1 mg in 1 kg or 1 μL in 1 L. Some comparisons could clarify these numbers: 1 ppm is 1 minute in 2 years; 1 cent of €10,000; 1 teaspoon of DDT spread over 2 hectares of land (20,000 m^2); 1 drop (0.05 mL) of vermouth in 50 L of gin, rather a dry martini cocktail.

What about a part per billion (10^{-9}), i.e., 1 μg in 1 kg? It is 1 minute in 2000 years; 1 person in the entire population of India; 1 medium-sized crouton in a 500-ton salad.

Toxicology: What Everyone Should Know. DOI: http://dx.doi.org/10.1016/B978-0-12-805348-5.00005-3

A part per trillion (10^{-12}) is 1 ng per 1 kg. It is 1 second in some 33,000 years; 1 square floor tile with sides of some 0.3 m on a kitchen floor twice the size of the Netherlands; 1 drop (0.05 mL) of vermouth in 50,000,000 L of gin, which is a very dry martini cocktail indeed.

We could go even lower to parts per quadrillion (10^{-15}), which stands for 1 pg per 1 kg. A ppq stands for one postage stamp on a letter the size of the states of California and Oregon combined; one human hair out of all the hair on all the heads of all the people in the world; 1.6 km on a journey of 170 light years (which is 1.6083×10^{15} km).

Now, these numbers give some context to concentration levels on which quite a few chemicals are regulated. Perhaps another way of giving perspective is figuring out the actual number of molecules we are dealing with when we talk about these levels. First, let's figure out how many molecules there are in an average tumbler filled with water.

To do this, we require Avogadro's constant, or the mole. Just like a dozen is 12 things of whatever, a mole is simply Avogadro's number of things, in chemistry that is atoms or molecules. The size of Avogadro's constant is quite large to say the least: 6.022×10^{23}. With this constant we can convert the directly measurable mass of, say, water into the actual number of water particles (H_2O), which we can't measure directly.

Let's assume we have 180 mL of pure water in the glass tumbler (Figure 5.1). That is 180 g of water, which amounts to 6.022×10^{24} molecules. So, 180 g/180 mL of water represents 10 moles of water molecules. A huge number. And the word huge doesn't even do justice to this number.

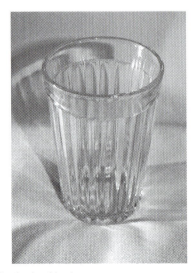

FIGURE 5.1 Picture of a classic table glass.

In fact, the number of water molecules in our glass closely outnumbers the amount of stars in the visible universe, which is estimated to be between 10^{22} and 10^{24} stars. That shows how many small molecules in fact are.

Adding sucrose (the normal sugar) to the pure water in our tumbler up to, say, 1 ppb would amount to adding just 0.18 μg of sucrose. That is, 3.167×10^{14} molecules of sugar. Again, this is a staggering amount of molecules, although the 0.18 μg could never be weighed in on a scale found in the average household kitchen. Specialized scientific scales are needed to be able to weigh such small amounts. Also, this amount of sugar in water is below our taste threshold, which is some 6 g of sucrose per liter, or roughly 1 g in our glass of water.

So, the world we are dealing with every day *and* the molecular world seem far apart in terms of mass and numbers of molecules, respectively. Although we can see the small and shiny sugar crystals we add to tea or coffee in the morning, the fact that these crystals are made up of so many discrete sucrose molecules baggers belief. Nevertheless, the macro of everyday life and the molecular of chemistry and toxicology are different expressions of the same thing.

Nevertheless, we are perceptive creatures and we can sense exposures to chemicals that are not agreeable to our physique, up to certain level of course. What toxicologists want to assess is at what levels of exposure we are safe, both on the short and the long term, and at what levels we need to take measures in order to lower or avoid exposures. Here, the natural

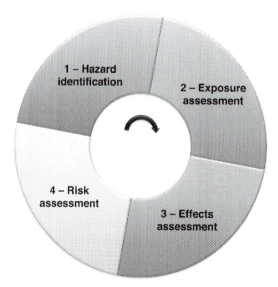

FIGURE 5.2 Picture of the classical risk assessment procedure.

sciences cannot provide all the answers. Because: how safe is safe enough? (Refer to Fig. 5.2.)

Now, the normal procedure in the field of toxicology is first to identify the hazard or hazards related to the chemical of choice. The hazard of a chemical is usually defined as the "inherent capability" to produce damage to organisms. Hazard identification encompasses gathering and evaluating data on the types of health effects or diseases that may be produced by a chemical at some dose. Additionally, exposure conditions under which environmental damage, injury, or disease will be produced need to be evaluated.

As soon as hazards are identified, the risks involved need to be assessed. A chemical that is hazardous to human health does not constitute a risk *unless* humans are exposed to it at a certain level. So the fact that hazards are known does not imply that we are by definition at risk. It all boils down to levels of exposure.

So the next step involves the appraisal of exposure levels. Not an easy task to perform. It involves estimating emissions from production in factories and household uses, and pathways and speeds of movement of a substance, e.g., through the air or water. Knowledge on its chemical and/or biological transformation and degradation is needed as well in order to obtain concentrations or doses to which human populations or environmental compartments are exposed.

It is obvious that exposure assessments are shrouded in uncertainties. The biggest unknowns are related to (1) the total emissions during production of the chemical, (2) the way it is used in society in all sorts of different products, and (3) the enormous geobiological variability across the globe such as climate, hydrology, geology, and biology, that influences the transport and transformation of the chemical.

Once we have a rough estimate of exposure, the effects related to such an exposure are mapped: the dose—response assessment. It is estimated what the relationship is between the level of exposure to a chemical (the dose), and the prevalence and severity of an effect or effects (the response). For that, a huge amount of information is required from experimental research with plants, test animals, and, very rarely, human volunteers. Also, population research (epidemiology) is done to tease out those effects that might be related to exposure to the chemical in question.

All these steps—(1) hazard identification, (2) exposure assessment, (3) effects assessment, (4) risk assessment—bring us to predicted or estimated no effect levels—NELs—for humans by dividing no observed adverse effect levels—NOAELs—found in laboratory animals or test systems using cells from animals or humans with some assessment factor, which usually lie in the range of 10–10,000. Assessment factors are numbers reflecting the estimated degree of uncertainty when experimental data from model systems (e.g., animal testing) are extrapolated to humans. Laboratory tests cover only a small part of the variety of responses that may occur in human populations. Extrapolation from experiments to humans involves numerous scientific uncertainties and assumptions. The higher the assessment factor, the lower the NEL, expressing a more cautious approach to the studied chemical. Lower NELs articulate the idea that more people are protected. The NELs are expressed in tolerable daily intakes—TDIs. The TDI is the daily intake of a chemical that, during the entire lifetime, appears to be without appreciable risk on the basis of all known facts at the time.

Overall, this brings us the risk characterization of the chemical. Now, taking this risk characterization process at face value, it seems that any exposure to any chemical should be as low as possible. In fact, avoiding all contact with chemicals seems the best option anyway. As we already pointed out, that is impossible and even dangerous. We are made of chemicals (there is much more to being human than that of course) and need food chemicals to stay alive and healthy. Chapter 4, Nature Knows Best—Chemicals From the Geobiological Sphere, dealt with that. Besides, all toxicological research would then immediately be superfluous.

To get to grips with chemical risk characterization, risk management comes into play, as other aspects than scientific analyses are required to balance the decision-making process. Overall the risk management process carries at least the following as shown in (Fig. 5.3).

In a nutshell, risk assessment asks "How risky is this chemical"?, whereas risk management asks "What shall we do about it"? This regulatory decision-making has become more developed and elaborate in the

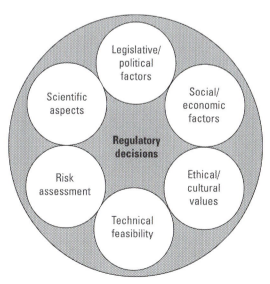

FIGURE 5.3 Risk management process (From U.S. Congress, Office of Technology Assessment, 1993. Researching Health Risks. U.S. Government Printing Office, Washington, DC.).

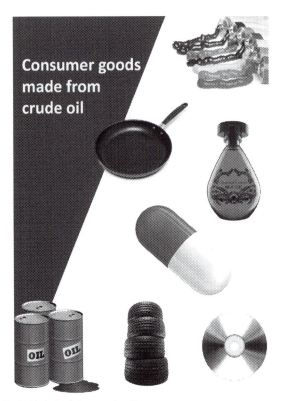

Consumer goods made from crude oil

FIGURE 5.4 Products derived from crude oil.

20th century. In fact, since the industrial revolution we have expanded our visible chemical surroundings, and this process accelerated in the previous century. Production processes that use crude oil as the basis for many different products, for instance, add to the mix of chemicals that we are "exposed" to such as pharmaceuticals, coatings, polymers, computers, pesticides, printer cartridges, toys, cell phones, tools, plastic film wrap for food. The list is almost endless. These products bring us all sorts of benefits and are traded off against any potential risks they might engender in mining, production, and use (Fig. 5.4).

The process of risk characterization brings together scientific knowledge, however limited considering the complexity, and value judgments that when joined together produces some kind of regulatory outcome. Some outcomes could be a safety standard for use in industry and at home, a ban because it is deemed too risky to produce and handle, further research on the chemical, and so on. And these scientific knowledge and value judgments are expressions of the culture we live, which could well be called precautionary.

RISK CHARACTERIZATION IN A PRECAUTIONARY CULTURE

Precaution seems a harmless, even prudent word of common usage and is ostensibly synonymous with prevention. However, they should be distinguished so as to understand precautionary culture and the way we view chemicals. The chemophobia we discussed in the last chapter is very much embedded in this precautionary culture.

Prevention means avoiding damage rather than remedying it after the damaging event. The damage to be avoided is clearly defined as resulting from a specific process or product in a chain of events: cutting one's finger in a food processor; injury caused by a car crash; food poisoning as a result of consuming food-borne pathogens such as *Salmonella enteritidis*, being exposed to chemicals when one paints the indoor woodwork; and so on. Thus, prevention entails putting in place measures to ensure, up to a certain point, that an already identified hazard cannot materialize, or to reduce its likelihood. Painters for instance can wear paint-spray facemasks during their indoor work as to prevent exposure to paint solvents.

Precaution on the other hand means an action taken in advance to protect against *possible* danger, failure, or injury. Precaution, as is understood nowadays, essentially takes prevention a critical step further, by deciding not to postpone physical, legal, or political interventions to prevent potential damage. This is done on the grounds that although scientific evidence of a potential hazard is limited or even absent, the hazard can never be excluded even though it might never materialize. We even have a legal principle of precaution, which states that "where there are threats of serious or irreversible damage, lack of full scientific certainty shall not be used as a reason for postponing cost-effective measures to prevent environmental degradation." It is also known as the triple-negative definition: *not* having scientific certainty is *not* a justification for *not* regulating, or just simply "when in doubt, don't."

In the risk characterization process described earlier, the move from hazard to risk is not really possible within the precautionary context. Scientific knowledge, no matter how elaborate, always carries limitations that make it impossible to characterize all the risks involved. Hazards of certain chemicals are then deemed enough to regulate on a precautionary basis.

Examples of precautionary regulation of certain chemicals are easy to give, especially for those chemicals that do not have an estimated NEL, and so no TDI can be estimated. That might be the case because toxicological knowledge is lacking, or if there are suspicions that the chemical involved could be carcinogenic, that will induce or promote cancer. We will discuss the latter more extensively in Chapter 6, Molecular Trepidations—The Linear Nonthreshold Model.

In Europe, zero-tolerance levels are in force for compounds without a TDI, meaning that banned chemicals should not be detected at all especially in food products. Obviously, analytical chemistry is not equipped to detect "nothing," so always has a minimum technical level to detect a chemical. That is for most chemicals in the range of parts per billion to parts per trillion.

Now, the first thing to consider is that molecules travel around the world in such a way that concentration levels of all chemicals are spread as evenly as possible. We know this phenomenon intimately—entropy; the progression to thermodynamic equilibrium, the heart of the second law of thermodynamics—from simple things. When sugar is added to a hot cup of coffee, the sugar dissolves and spreads evenly throughout the coffee. What you will never observe is that the just dissolved sugar suddenly returns to a lump of undissolved sugar at the bottom of your morning brew. Entropy drives the inexorable diffusion (spread) of chemicals throughout this world. The fact that we are literally stardust (again, and much more than that) could not be a better description of this diffusion process operative in the cosmos!

Second, some chemicals that are regarded as worthy of regulation—a pesticide, an antibiotic, an antifouling agent on ship's hulls, and so on—are explicitly regarded as synthetic, man-made, so if you find these in the environment or food, then an installed ban is easily enforced and by default deemed as effective. When it is found it has been illegally used; once people stop using the chemical it will simply disappear because of dilution and degradation. So the Nettles family in the beginning of this chapter have to face the consequences of their illegal labor. The detection of some breakdown products (metabolites) of the banned drug furazolidone is enough indication for the competent authorities to conclude that they used an illegal drug in their cows. But is that true?

We already pointed out in the previous chapter that the so-called synthetic chemicals might very well have natural sources as well. This has been shown extensively for organohalogens, which were once regarded as exclusively man-made. So what about furazolidone and its marker metabolite 3-amino-2-oxazolidinone (AOZ)?

The trust competent authorities place in such marker molecules is misplaced, as history shows. In 2009 there was an increased incidence in Belgium in the detection of semicarbazide (SEM), a marker molecule for the banned antibiotic nitrofurazone, in the freshwater prawns *Macrobrachium rosenbergii*. Nitrofurazone belongs to same class of antibiotics as furazolidone.

This was in contrast with all other European countries where no significant increase in SEM positive samples was reported. A possible explanation for this phenomenon was that at request of the Belgian Federal Agency for the Safety of the Food Chain, all approved laboratories were asked to analyses complete prawns (meat and shell) for the presence of metabolites of nitrofurans from December 17, 2004, onward. This procedure is not common in other countries, as only the meat is sampled.

SEM as a marker for nitrofurazone was already questionable as it was found that certain food production and packaging circumstances resulted in the formation of SEM. Experimental research later showed that crustaceans produce SEM at varying concentrations. The source of SEM, now positively identified as a natural metabolite, is unknown as of yet.

Clearly, SEM cannot be used as a marker molecule for the illegal use of nitrofurazone. The purported legal link between the presence of SEM and the prohibited use of nitrofurazone is broken. The fact that SEM is a natural metabolite in crustaceans rules out the possibility to track illegal nitrofurazone use through the use of SEM as a marker.

The idea that an unambiguous causal link can be made between the detection of some banned chemical and illegality in food production is overall untenable. Chloramphenicol, another banned and purported man-made antibiotic, roused quite the food scare at the beginning of the 21st century. Here as well, presence was regarded straightforwardly as the result of illegal use. However, unsurprisingly, it has been found as a natural component in plant material, which is used as animal feed through which it is transferred to animal tissue. This example is quite similar to the issue of the natural background of polybrominated diphenyl ethers (PBDEs) we discussed in the previous chapter.

Mother Nature thus amply supplies us with chemicals that we rather not have in our environment and our food. We even try to organize this by law, which clearly she doesn't abide by. And although we haven't found a natural source yet for AOZ, the marker molecule for furazolidone, history and chemistry learns that we most likely will. The question then arises why we would have zero-tolerance laws in the first place? Is it about hazards and the exposures thereto, or eradicating illegal use of chemicals (which does happen), or perhaps something else? It seems clear that the hazards-discourse so favored by regulators and politicians is the goal of choice, and the eradication of illegal use piggybacks thereon.

PRECAUTION AND ETHICS

In order to gauge the depth of this, we have to go back to the risk characterization of chemicals. This seems a very straightforward process that neatly separates science from regulation. But things are never that simple as we already have seen. We live in an age where safety should be maximized and if chemicals are suspected of hazards of especially a carcinogenic kind, everything must be done to ensure their absence from the environment to which we are exposed. That is the precautionary response: "when in doubt, leave it out."

So, when reviewing the risk characterization process, assessment factors can be dialed up as to make the NELs as low as possible. There is even a term for that: ALARA—as low as reasonably achievable. But reasonableness is known for its elasticity, that might be stretched to even the idea that some chemicals simply should not exist, expressed as zero tolerance.

As the assessment factors are an expression of the uncertainty surrounding the scientific process of uncovering the risks of exposure to chemicals, precautionary culture feeds off this uncertainty. Precautionary politics in principle is never satisfied with research showing that no adverse effects have been reported at a certain level of exposure, the basis for an NEL. As "absence of evidence" is not considered to be "evidence of absence," proponents of precaution stress that adverse effects in spite of all the available evidence may yet arise in the (far) future. Our safety, security, health, and longevity should be guaranteed by science.

In precautionary culture then, science finds itself between a rock and a hard place: a very high level of skepticism with regard to what science cannot and should not do—give a chemical a clean bill of health—goes hand in hand with a very high level of confidence regarding what science is supposed to deliver—give a chemical a clean bill of health. So, science is never free from the culture in which it has grown from a scientific discipline into an overarching advisory role for society and politics on what is safe and what is not in the "chemical world." And of course, very few things are really safe, as with precautionary culture we have stepped into a realm of perceived *absolute* safety.

So, if even science cannot guarantee our chemical safety, then regulation should do the rest. And that it has done, or so it seems. It should therefore not be surprising that we are bombarded with chemical scares through press releases, newspaper items, new and widely advertised more stringent laws, and so on. We have become a scared people, tying in nicely with the chemophobia we discussed previously.

That leaves us with the one question, namely how to value risks of chemicals exposures, including those chemicals we do not want and we have banned from our environment to which we are exposed to daily. A number of issues are encapsulated in this not so simple question.

For one, science knows quite a bit of many different chemicals, and we should take that knowledge seriously, but *not* as definitive. Things change and so does science. The more we know about the chemical and toxicological world, the more we are baffled by its complexity. That brings us to the second point.

We are adaptable people. That is what we do: we adapt. As said earlier, we are exposed to thousands and thousands of different chemicals every day and we adapt to those chemicals, including the carcinogenic stuff we naturally find in our environment. And the better we can adapt, the better our health is. In fact, we "train" ourselves through that massively diverse exposure: eating healthy is related to a diversified diet, and that means more chemicals, not less.

Third, those chemicals that are regulated simply caught our attention, especially if these chemicals are produced industrially. It also shows that we regulate the so-called simple stuff, the chemicals we can "see." We simply ignore the rest, and for good reason. There is simply too much to research and regulate. That the simple regulated stuff sometimes surprises us through Mother Nature should *not* be surprising. And then we lose interest. Dioxins were all the rage in the 1970s and 1980s as it was advertised as the most toxic man-made chemical ever. And then we discovered natural sources of this not so toxic compound after all, even in ourselves. Very few people discuss dioxins nowadays.

Fourth, precaution has made us very wary of anything chemical, paradoxically combined with a lack of general knowledge of the chemical. That drives many different research efforts and very public displays of force, such as the killing of all the cows on the Nettles farm, which in fact is an actual case that we have anonymized.

The last aspect is material for our next chapter. We so much fear carcinogenic chemicals that we evaluate them separately in comparison to all other chemicals that are not regarded as carcinogenic, at least as far as we know. We think that every single molecule of a carcinogenic chemical could cause cancer. Whether or not that is even remotely true we will delve into next. Nevertheless, that is how we regulate such chemicals into purported oblivion. And again and again, we find reality opposing that misplaced legalistic instinct.

REFERENCES AND FURTHER READING

Berendsen, B., Stolker, L., de Jong, J., Nielen, M., Tserendorj, E., Sodnomdarjaa, R., et al., 2010. Evidence of natural occurrence of the banned antibiotic chloramphenicol in herbs and grass. Anal. Bioanal. Chem. 397, 1955–1963.

Berendsen, B., Pikkemaat, M., Römkens, P., Wegh, R., van Sisseren, M., Stolker, L., et al., 2013. Occurrence of chloramphenicol in crops through natural production by bacteria in soil. J. Agric. Food Chem. 61, 4004–4010.

Hanekamp, J.C., 2015. *Utopia and Gospel: Unearthing the Good News in Precautionary Culture*. PhD Thesis. Tilburg University, ISBN 978-90-823225-0-7.

Hanekamp, J.C., Frapporti, G., Olieman, K., 2003. Chloramphenicol, food safety and precautionary thinking in Europe. Environ. Liabil. 6, 209–221.

Hanekamp, J.C., Kwakman, J., Olieman, K., 2011. Crossing the ecological threshold of scientific analysis, natural chemicals and global trade. Anal. Bioanal. Chem. 399, 2223–2224.

Hoenicke, K., Gatermann, R., Hartig, L., Mandix, M., Otte, S., 2004. Formation of semicarbazide (SEM) in food by hypochlorite treatment—is SEM a specific marker for nitrofurazone abuse? Food. Addit. Contam. 21, 526–537.

Purves, D., Augustine, G.J., Fitzpatrick, D., Hall, W.C., LaMantia, A.-S., McNamara, J.O., et al., 2004. Neuroscience, Third ed. Sinauer Associates, Inc, MA.

Saari, L., Peltonen, K., 2004. Novel source of semicarbazide: levels of semicarbazide in cooked crayfish samples determined by LC/MS/MS. Food Addit. Contam. 21, 825–832.

See <http://www.accessdata.fda.gov/CMS_IA/importalert_1153.html> (accessed 23.06.16).

See <http://www.waterontheweb.org/resources/conversiontables.html> (accessed 23.06.16).

See <www.unep.org/Documents.multilingual/Default.asp?DocumentID = 78&ArticleID = 1163&l = en> (accessed 23.06.16).

U.S. Congress, Office of Technology Assessment, 1993. Researching Health Risks. U.S. Government Printing Office, Washington, DC.

Van Leeuwen, C.J., Vermeire, T.G., 2007. Risk Assessment of Chemicals, An Introduction, Second ed. Springer, The Netherlands.

Van Poucke, C., Detaverniert, C., Wille, M., Kwakman, J., Sorgeloos, P., Van Peteghem, C., 2011. Investigation into the possible natural occurrence of semicarbazide in *Macrobrachium rosenbergii* Prawns. J. Agric. Food Chem. 59, 2107−2112.

Chapter 6

Molecular Trepidations—The Linear Nonthreshold Model

The Golden Ratio (sectio aurea) has fascinated us from antiquity onward. The first clear definition was given around 300 BC by Euclid of Alexandria: "A straight line is said to have been cut in extreme and mean ratio when, as the whole line is to the greater segment, so is the greater to the lesser." In other words, if a line of length AB is intersected at point C so that the ratio of AB/AC is the same as AC/CB, then the line is cut in Golden Ratio. The precise value of the Golden Ratio (the ratio of AC to CB) is the never-ending, never-repeating so-called irrational number 1.6180339887... also known as phi (φ; see Fig. 6.1). Patterns in nature, such as the spiral symmetry seen in the sunflower and the nautilus shell apparently representing the Golden Ratio, are usually regarded as beautiful. The question of course is whether this fascinating geometrical curiosity is actually an intrinsic part of the world we live in or that we impress this Ratio on nature. This conundrum is similarly found in toxicology. Models to assess the relation between dose (concentration) and response are usually represented in a manageable and forthright way, such as a straight line. Chemicals are regarded as cancer causing (carcinogenic): just one molecule thereof is thought to be potentially enough to wreak havoc with a person's health in the long run. And for that reason, the scientific community devised a toxicological model, the linear nonthreshold (LNT) model, to set the required toxicological standards for such chemicals. In this chapter we will assess that model and see whether science can deliver what the model seems to promise: a world where chemical—carcinogenic risks can be overcome. To put it candidly, might the model not be a straightjacket, which research is forced into so as to "obey" the predetermined model.

CORPORA NON AGUNT NISI FIXATA—AGENTS ONLY WORK WHEN THEY ARE BOUND

In the previous chapter, we discussed the valuation of risks as a result of chemicals exposure, keeping in mind that exposure to chemicals is fundamentally unavoidable. The irrefutable merging of science and precautionary

Toxicology: What Everyone Should Know. DOI: http://dx.doi.org/10.1016/B978-0-12-805348-5.00006-5

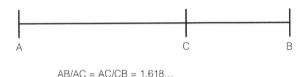

$$AB/AC = AC/CB = 1.618...$$

FIGURE 6.1 Golden Ratio.

policymaking was one issue we discussed as an expression of the culture we all live in.

What we only hinted at was the dose−response relationship between chemicals exposure and observed effects. This dose−response relationship is essential as it expresses the well-known empirical observation that different dose levels result in different effects in organisms such as us. Very roughly summarizing dose−response: "small" doses—no or small effects; "large" doses—large effects. And of course, many intermediate doses and responses can be envisaged and scrutinised.

This ballpark estimation obviously raises very important questions: How small is small and how large is large? Are effects immediately visible after exposure? Can doses be so small that there can be no effects: a threshold value? What about long-term effects of small doses: could they be dangerous after all? These are all questions to which the field of toxicology tries to formulate answers to.

However, a particular group of chemicals are regarded as an exception namely the carcinogenic (cancer-causing) chemicals. Specifically, the genotoxic carcinogens—compounds that interact with the hereditary material such as DNA—are thought to be operative on organisms at any dose level except zero. So, even one molecule of such chemicals is thought to be able to cause disease over a certain period of time.

This chapter discusses precaution within the scientific framework of toxicological research. As we will see, this precautionary approach seems attractive, yet can never deliver its protective health perspectives it advertises. In order to add flesh and bone to this claim, we need to go back in time.

During the fin de siècle, it was Paul Ehrlich (1854−1915) who made many discoveries in the fields of physiology and medicine and gave them secure footing. His work influenced research not only in both fields but also in toxicology in multiple ways that still stand today. According to Ehrlich, chemotherapy should be based on the principle of selective affinity. In his own words:

> *The whole field is governed by a simple, I might even say natural, principle. If the law is true in chemistry that* corpora non agunt nisi liquida, *then for chemotherapy the principle is true that* corpora non agunt nisi fixata. *When applied to the special case in point, this means that parasites are killed only by those substances for which they have a certain affinity, by virtue of which these are fixed by the parasites.*

The first Latin phrase in Ehrlich's statement—*corpora non agunt nisi liquida*; agents will not work unless dissolved—is from Paracelsus (1493–1541) and conveys the notion that for any activity—chemical, biochemical, biological—a compound must be in (a watery) solution. The molecules, atoms, or ions must not be bound to any great extent to themselves, that is, in a crystalline or amorphous solid.

Paracelsus' insight forms an important milestone in man's understanding of the chemical activity of any compound, including its effects on biological structures. It is as valid today as it was more than 400 years ago. Nevertheless, it does not give us any information on *how* the biological effects are mediated. Ehrlich's postulate, the second Latin phrase in the above quote which is an iteration on Paracelsus's, tries to fill the gap: substances do not exert their biological activity unless they become attached. The question of course is attached to what?

Ehrlich's observations on the binding of dyes to proteins and, more importantly, the distinct differences in binding affinities led to his "side chain" theory. Chemical substances become bound to specific receptors (proteins), which are located at the cellular level and act as a link between the compounds and the reactive tissue. This attachment to the "chemoreceptor"—represented clearly in the lock and key model—was originally considered by him to be so firm as to be practically irreversible. This proved to be false. The binding of a receptor with the active substance might also result in dissociable complexes. Nevertheless, his theory on binding of chemicals to endogenous "receptors" and its biochemical effects on organisms are the bread and butter of pharmacology and toxicology.

THE GOLDEN RATIO…

These insights of Ehrlich, and many other scientists after him, led to the understanding of the interaction of chemicals with organisms including humans. That obviously is the task of science: unearthing the hidden structure of reality. Conversely, *imposing* order on said found structure similarly is a process well known in the history of science. This may also result in tunnel vision.

As introduced at the start of this chapter, the Golden Ratio is an age-old example of order either found in nature or impressed on nature. The Golden Ratio is expressed, among others, by the so-called Fibonacci sequence. It is a sequence of numbers—0, 1, 1, 2, 3, 5, 8, 13, 21, 34, 55, 89, 144, etc.—comprising of an addition of the two previous numbers. In this series, any number in the sequence (larger than 3) divided by its predecessor has an approximate value of 1.618 (phi; φ). One visual representation of the Golden Ratio in geometry is the line division as described by Euclid (see above). Another is the so-called golden spiral. This is a logarithmic spiral whose growth factor is φ (Fig. 6.2).

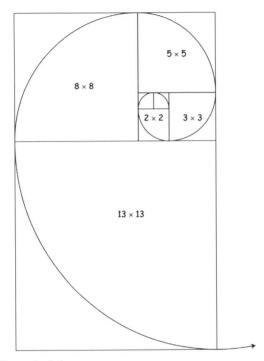

FIGURE 6.2 Fibonacci spiral.

The Golden Ratio purportedly is found in many natural environments. For example, the nautilus shell usually is put forward as *the* example that expresses this Golden Ratio. Optimal seedpacking in sunflower heads seem to follow the Golden Ratio. The ordering of leaves of plants seems to follow the Golden Ratio as well (Fig. 6.3).

Vitruvian man of Leonardo da Vinci is drawn according to the Ratio. Indeed, even a man's arm seems to follow phi. We even impose phi on ratios of the human face most of us would find attractive, that is to say aesthetically pleasing. Subsequently, we state that such a face having this ratio *is* attractive. Thereby, phi is equated with beauty (Fig. 6.4).

But is it true that the Golden Ratio is an unwavering mathematical characteristic of our world? That is a question not easily answered; finding the Golden Ratio in natural phenomena and organisms does not solve the puzzle whether the Golden Ration is intrinsically part of nature. (In fact, it is a metaphysical question, which the empirical sciences could not possibly hope to answer.) More to the point, we are able to *impose* the Golden Ratio. For example, looking more closely at the famous nautilus shell, it does not seem conform to this ratio, although these shells vary in spiral form and size.

Occasionally, we seem to impose order rather than discover it in the structure of reality. What about toxicology? Do we impose some form of

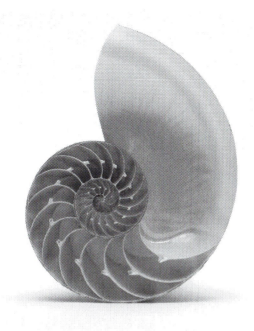

FIGURE 6.3 The nautilus shell.

order without paying attention to the order that in fact is? Linearity as frequently applied to explain toxicological results seems to be an example of a modern Golden Ratio of sorts.

... AND THE LNT MODEL

To give an idea of the importance of linearity, we here show an example thereof that is crucial in pharmacology. A hyperbolic relation between substrate concentration and the enzymatic rate usually describes enzymatic reactions. When the chemical that is converted by the enzyme is more abundant, the reaction rate will increase. Obviously, there is a maximum to that, and that is at the point where the substrate chemicals occupy all individual enzymes. As a result, the reaction rate cannot increase anymore (Fig. 6.5).

From this graph, as is shown, a maximal reaction rate (v_{max}) and a K_m (the concentration needed to reach half v_{max}) can be obtained. These parameters describe the characteristics of the enzymatic reaction.

In order to determine these parameters more accurately, one usually linearizes the hyperbolic relation, also known as the Lineweaver−Burke transformation. Herein we plot the inverse substrate concentration vs the inverse rate. Having done this, it is easy to read off the v_{max} on the y-axis and the K_m on the x-axis (Fig. 6.6). Remarkably, the lowest substrate concentrations

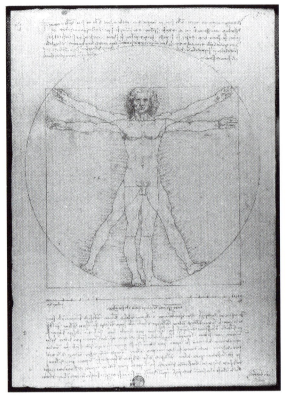

FIGURE 6.4 Vitruvian man.

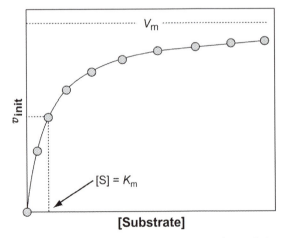

FIGURE 6.5 Hyperbolic relation between substrate concentration and the enzymatic rate. *From Enzyme Kinetics: Catalysis & Control: A Reference of Theory and Best-Practice Methods.*

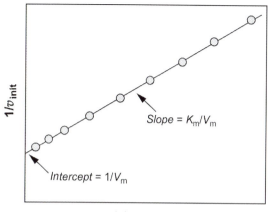

1/[Substrate]

FIGURE 6.6 Lineweaver–Burke plot. *From Enzyme Kinetics: Catalysis & Control: A Reference of Theory and Best-Practice Methods.*

(where the lowest rates are measured) are the most difficulty to acquire, yet carry the most weight in determining the slope of the line, and thereby the enzymatic parameters.

A comparable linearization of a hyperbolic relationship is found in pharmacology. This linearization concerns the concentration of a drug vs the percentage of receptors occupied by the drug *or* the concentration of a drug vs the effect caused by receptor occupancy. However, in this case, linearization is obtained via plotting the logarithm of the concentration of the drug to either the receptor occupancy or the effect thereof (Fig. 6.7).

Linearity facilitates the readout of the 50% effects/response. However, this linearization occurs only between 20% and 80% of receptor occupancy or receptor effect. The most fundamental processes—i.e., enzyme kinetics

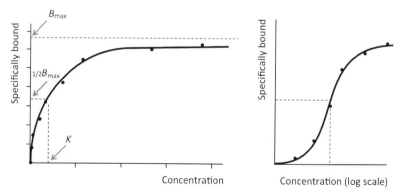

FIGURE 6.7 Specific binding plotted against concentration.

and receptor functions—are reduced to linear relationships, albeit with discipline-specific differences. Thereby linearity seems to not only have a normal reductionist function—science cannot research everything and anything—but is subsequently understood, either inadvertently or explicitly, as the underlying and all too real rule of thumb of pharmacology and toxicology. This is a gross simplification of the nature of the observed and studied phenomena and has all sorts of consequences.

One unequivocal corollary of the linear approach is that any chemical/drug seems to be able to exert only one effect that increases with the dose. Linearity thus imposes its order on the understanding of chemical compounds as either "good" or "bad." And both can only be described as "graded" depending on dose, whereby the classical Paracelsus axiom is a priori infused with either of the two understandings of chemical effects. The one excludes the other.

Within this perspective, genotoxic carcinogens and ionizing radiation are regarded as particularly and specifically bad up to the individual molecular/photonic level. The classical stance on the risk of ionizing radiation is this: "Complexities notwithstanding, the genetic damage done, however felt and however measured, is roughly proportional to the total mutation rate." ... "Any radiation is genetically undesirable, since any radiation induces harmful mutations. Further, all presently available scientific information leads to the conclusion that the genetic harm is proportional to the total dose .... This tells us that a radiation dose of 2X must be presumed to be twice as harmful as a radiation dose of X." This line of reasoning has been broadened to chemical compounds. Consequently, two molecules of carcinogens would increase the risk of cancer by a factor of two.

But, what kind of scientific experiment(s) would suffice to show that such a notion is indeed tenable? The answer is simple: no experiment would actually be possible to causally connect exposure to one molecule or two and the increase of cancer risk.

Despite this fatal flaw in the logic of this model, the calculation of cancer risks requires some causal model of dose–response, data on exposure (or dose), and probability of response. The subsequent numerals are developed on the empirically unverifiable *assumption* of proportionality between very low dose and probability of response (the risk): any non-zero exposure has a non-zero probability of causing cancer. This model, obviously, becomes non-linear at higher doses because it cannot exceed one: it is a cumulative probability function of lifetime cancer deaths. This is the classical LNT postulate.

And from this classical postulate a number of conundrums arise. For one, there is an absurd quality to the notion that every single or photon with genotoxic attributes could be unreservedly detrimental to human health. Already in 1996, Goldman noted the palpable incongruity of the LNT model when he linearly calculated the increased risk of cancer, because of increased cosmic ionizing radiation, if the entire world population would add a 1-inch lift to their shoes (*sic*):

As an extreme extrapolation, consider that everyone on Earth adds a 1-inch lift to their shoes for just 1 year. The resultant very small increase in cosmic ray dose (it doubles for every 2000 m in altitude), multiplied by the very large population of the Earth, would yield a collective dose large enough to kill about 1500 people with cancer over the next 50 years. Of course no epidemiological confirmation of this increment could ever be made, and although the math is approximately correct, the underlying assumptions should be questioned. Most of the environmental risks we now face from present or proposed activities probably are of this magnitude, and many of our policies say that prudence requires us to reduce these small values even further. We do not seem to have a realistic process whereby we can uniformly both protect the public health and avoid seemingly frivolous prevention schemes.

Goldman, despite his flippant exemplar, does describe the basic assumptions of the LNT model properly. What is more, a dose of various carcinogens associated with a *de minimis* ("de minimis non curat lex"—"the law does not concern itself with trifles") risk of cancer, i.e., <1 cancer (disease)/million/lifetime exposure (also known as the maximum tolerable risk level; MTR), would imply an exposure to many *trillions of carcinogenic molecules* each day and during a human life span. This value approaches and at times exceeds some 18 orders of magnitude greater than a single carcinogenic molecule. That gives pause to think.

An example will give more depth to this notion. Aflatoxins (Af) B_1, B_2, G_1, and G_2 are mycotoxins that are produced by three moulds of the *Aspergillus* species: *A. flavus*, *A. parasiticus*, and *A. nomius*. These moulds contaminate plants and plant products that are used for animal feed and food products for human consumption. Aflatoxin B_1 is the most frequent one present in contaminated samples and aflatoxins B_2, G_1, and G_2 are generally not reported in the absence of aflatoxin B_1. Most of the toxicological data relate to aflatoxin B_1. Dietary intake of aflatoxins arises mainly from contamination of maize and groundnuts and their products such as peanut butter.

In Europe, the maximum regulatory level in certain foods (such as almonds, pistachios, and apricot kernels), intended for direct human consumption or use as an ingredient in foodstuffs, is between 2 and 12 ppb. AfB_1 is regulated separately at 2 ppb in Europe, whereas the sum total is set at 10 ppb. In the United States, AfB_1 is not regulated separately: a sum standard is set at 20 ppb. Choosing 10 ppb would roughly amount to 1.928×10^{16} aflatoxin B_1 molecules per kilogram of a certain contaminated food product. And 20 ppb would be double that amount of molecules: 3.856×10^{16}.

Thus, exposure to aflatoxin B_1, or any other of the aflatoxins, even with a limited consumption of contaminated foods, by far exceeds the LNT exposure restriction of a single molecule, if one wants to avoid risks of cancer as a result of exposure to genotoxic carcinogens. Indeed, the joint FAO/WHO Expert Committee on Food Additives (JECFA) concluded in their risk assessment on aflatoxins, on the assumption that at very low levels of exposure the linear dose–response curve holds, that "reducing the hypothetical standard from 20 to 10 μg/kg yields a drop in the estimated population risk of approximately 2 additional cancers/year per 10^9 (billion; authors) people."

CONSEQUENCES OF A MISCONCEPTION—SOME CONCLUDING THOUGHTS

The first thing that sticks out in this discussion on the LNT model is that once we convert ppm, ppb, or even ppt—milligrams, micrograms, and nanograms—into actual numbers of molecules involved, digits go from quite small to astronomically large. This simply underlines the notion already touched upon earlier that molecules are extremely small things.

And although it seems quite praiseworthy of societies to want to increase certain safety standards by trying to lower exposure in order to protect public health, from a molecular point of view such a move looks completely different and far less impressive; quite the contrary. Regulating on the ppt-, ppq-level or even pushing towards zero-tolerance in order to protect public health seems profound, but that profundity vanishes into thin air once actual numbers of molecules are considered. No wonder that toxicologists and regulators never took on Avogadro's number; all micro-managerial safety-policy efforts seem futile in light thereof. The example given above shows that both standards—10 and 20 μg/kg— represent astronomical numbers of molecules that are very far removed from the hypothetical one molecule. This is specifically noteworthy when considering compounds such as aflatoxins, or any other genotoxic carcinogen or ionizing photon. Then, so the model goes, every "hit" by a molecule or photon counts.

That brings us to the following aspect. Linearity underscores the absolute dichotomy between good and bad in chemical exposure. But this is the result of taking the model too seriously. Linearity is hardly a descriptive reality in toxicology and physiology at all. Nevertheless, it functions as a prescriptive reduction of both. It thus seems that in toxicology we have our own Golden Ratio. We seemingly cannot do without prescriptive structures, despite the severe limitations those engender subsequently, both theoretically and experimentally.

Therefore, linear approaches may easily generate the *reification fallacy*. Abstractions are very useful—understanding certain physiological processes as linear is an example of such an abstraction—and are of themselves harmless when we keep in mind that we *are* abstracting. However, we run into severe problems when we think of abstractions as if they were actual realities themselves, thereby "reifying" (objectifying) them. Worse, when we think of the abstractions as somehow more real than the concrete realities from which they have been abstracted, then we find ourselves in a real pickle.

And obviously, there is a more thoroughgoing outlook within toxicology and pharmacology, which attempts to incorporate the complexity that is our interaction with the chemical outside world. And that we already described

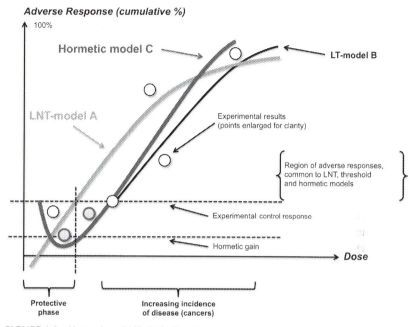

FIGURE 6.8 Hormesis vs LNT (including the threshold model).

earlier: we adapt. We are not passive recipients of all those trillions of carcinogenic molecules that might inflict chaos in our physiology.

Indeed, we seem to thrive on those toxicological insults that test our physiology within the bounds of our homeostasis, the dynamic balance between health and disease. And the ability to adapt suspends the purported and self-placed boundary between "good" and "bad" chemicals. Increasing scientific knowledge on low-dose exposures to chemicals, including those chemicals we ideally like to ban from our sphere of living, indicates that the dose—response curve is not linear but J-shaped. This J-shape is usually referred to as hormetic or biphasic and denotes some adaptive response of the exposed organism. Hormesis is in many ways the physiological equivalent of the philosophical notion that "what won't kill you, will make you strong." Hormesis is best described as an adaptive response to low levels of stress or damage (from for example chemicals or radiation), resulting in enhanced robustness of some physiological systems for a finite period.

For example, heavy metals such as mercury prompt synthesis of proteins called metallothioneins that remove toxic metals from circulation and probably also protect cells against potentially DNA-damaging free radicals produced through normal metabolism. Conversely, low concentrations of antitumor agents commonly enhance the proliferation of the human tumor cells, in a manner that is fully consistent with the hormetic dose—response relationship.

High concentrations push the organism beyond the limits of kinetic (distribution, biotransformation, or excretion) or dynamic (adaptation, repair, or reversibility) recovery. This is a classical toxicological object of research usually required as a result of public and regulatory concerns, whereby hormetic responses are by default regarded as irrelevant, or even contrary to policy interests, and therefore unlooked for (Fig. 6.8).

Overall, the biphasic, hormetic, performance between organisms and chemicals redefines the concept of "pollution" and "contamination." It questions the premise that "pollutants," "toxins," are categorically bad, as suggested by the language used. This is innovative because modern food safety, environmental and public health legislation is built in large part, due to the reductionist linear models, on the moral dichotomies of good vs evil, clean vs dirty, natural vs unnatural. Chemical substances are neither bad nor good; they are both depending on exposure levels and adaptive responses from the exposed organisms.

When regulatory agencies focus exclusively on the harmful side of exposure at low doses, which is not empirically defined but simply assumed and thus ignoring its potential beneficial effects, it negates the statutory mandate to *adequately protect human health*. Thus, the very reason for being conservative, in the classical precautionary sense, fails to protect; quite the contrary.

Our ability to adapt is the fundamental evolutionary advantage we absolutely require to survive a hostile chemical and physical environment. Indeed, we require this hostility to our healthy advantage within homeostatic limits. We have been duped by the fool's gold that is the linear worldview.

REFERENCES AND FURTHER READING

Bast, A., Hanekamp, J.C., 2014. "You can't always get what you want"—linearity as the Golden Ratio of toxicology. Dose Response 12 (4), 664–672.

Calabrese, E.J., Baldwin, L.A., 2003. Toxicology rethinks its central belief. Hormesis demands a reappraisal of the way risks are assessed. Nature. 421, 691–692.

Commission Regulation (EU) No 165/2010 of 26 February 2010 amending Regulation (EC) No 1881/2006 setting maximum levels for certain contaminants in foodstuffs as regards aflatoxins. Official J. Eur. Union L50: 8–12.

Committee on Genetic Effects of Atomic Radiation, 1956. Genetic effects of atomic radiation. Science 123, 1157–1164.

Dale, H. (Ed.), 1960. The Collected Papers of Paul Ehrlich. Pergamon Press, London, Oxford, New York, Paris.

European food Safety Authority, 2007. Opinion of the scientific panel on contaminants in the food chain on a request from the commission related to the potential increase of consumer health risk by a possible increase of the existing maximum levels for aflatoxins in almonds, hazelnuts and pistachios and derived products. EFSA J. 446, 1–127.

Garner, B.A. (Ed.), 2009. Black's Law Dictionary, ninth ed. Thomson Reuters, St. Paul, MN.

Goldman, M., 1996. Cancer risk of low-level exposure. Science 271, 1821–1822.

Health Council of the Netherlands. 2010. Guideline to the classification of carcinogenic compounds. Guide for classifying compounds in terms of their carcinogenic properties, and for assessing their genotoxicity. Health Council of the Netherlands, publication no. A10/07E, The Hague, The Netherlands.

Kaiser, J., 2003. Sipping from a poisoned chalice. Science 320, 376–378.

Kaufmann, S.H.E., 2008. Paul Ehrlich: founder of chemotherapy. Nat. Rev. Drug. Discov. 7, 373.

Kourtis, N., Nikoletopoulou, V., Tavernarakis, N., 2012. Small heat-shock proteins protect from heat-stroke-associated neurodegeneration. Nature. 490, 213–221.

Livio, M., 2002. The Golden Ratio: The Story of Phi, the World's Most Astonishing Number. Broadway Books, New York, NY.

Nelson, D.L., Cox, M.M., 2012. Lehninger Principles of Biochemistry, *sixth ed.* W.H. Freeman, New York, NY.

Otsuki, T., Wilson, J.S., Sewadeh, M., 2001. Saving two in a billion: quantifying the trade effect of European food safety standards on African exports. Food. Policy. 26, 495–514.

Prokopakis, E.P., Vlastos, I.M., Picavet, V.A., Nolst Trenite, G., Thomas, R., Cingi, C., et al., 2013. The Golden Ratio in facial symmetry. Rhinology. 51 (1), 18–21.

See <http://www.inchem.org/documents/jecfa/jecmono/v040je16.htm> (accessed 27.09.16).

Sharp, J., 2002. Spirals and the Golden Section. Nexus Network J. 4 (1), 59–82.

Westphal, U., 1971. Steroid–Protein Interactions. Springer-Verlag, Berlin, Heidelberg, New York.

Who Food Additives Series 40, 1998.

Chapter 7

"The Policy of Truth" — Anchoring Toxicology in Regulation

Lecturing on pharmacotherapy to medical students at the University of Maastricht is an enthralling task. During the fifth year of their study, the students follow an internship of several weeks at a practice of a family doctor. The students are asked to describe a case they encounter in which the patient receives polypharmacy treatment. The patient, frequently an elderly patient, receives multiple drugs for various diseases. The student is then requested to discuss the case with the supervising family doctor and the local pharmacist. Discussion on the action of the drugs, the choice for certain medication, the side effects, interactions between the drugs, and so on are subsequently debated between the students and the lecturer at the university. Indeed a fascinating task.

A frequently occurring observation is that the multitude of drugs may lead to what is known as "anticholinergic accumulation." It appears that many drugs inhibit the cholinergic system. This even holds for drugs without an evident anticholinergic action. Elderly people have a more fragile blood—brain barrier and the accumulation of these anticholinergic drugs in polypharmacy may lead to cognitive impairment. Drugs used for sleep, antiemetics, urinary incontinence, and also respiratory drugs, antidepressants, antipsychotics, and antiparkinson agents may add to this anticholinergic effect. Also over-the-counter, cold and flu remedies contribute to this effect. This seems to be a large problem in the steadily older growing population; however, no safety regulations seem applicable.

Toxicology and regulatory health and safety standards play a major role in the life of citizens of the Western World. Toxicology seems to be anchored in policymaking and regulation randomly. What kind of interaction takes place as to define, apply, and refine regulatory standards?

FROM TOXICOLOGY TO LEGISLATION

Articles on scientific failures always mention the example of thalidomide which is also known under several trade names like Softenon (in the

Toxicology: What Everyone Should Know. DOI: http://dx.doi.org/10.1016/B978-0-12-805348-5.00007-7

Netherlands and Belgium) or Contergan (in Germany). The thalidomide disaster occurred in the 1950s. The sleeping and tranquilizing drug caused the birth of thousands of children with malformations.

After the introduction in the 1950s, thalidomide seemed a miracle drug. The sleeping drug was very effective in alleviating morning sickness in pregnant women. Moreover it seemed strikingly safe. It did not suppress breathing, something which was associated with older sleeping drugs.

Around 1960, some publications caused concern. The first report was that upon long-term use, the drug possibly caused nerve damage. Shortly after the introduction of thalidomide, the number of children with phocomelia increased, a severe condition in which the limbs of children were shortened or were even completely absent.

In Germany the drug was widely used. The Department of Pediatrics of the University of Hamburg did not have a single patient with phocomelia between 1949 and 1959. But in 1959, there was one patient; in 1960, 30; and in 1961, not less than 154 were identified. At that time, a smart German pediatrician, Dr. Lenz suspected a causal link between the use of thalidomide by pregnant women and the occurrence of phocomelia. It appeared that the use of the drug by the mother between the third and eighth week of pregnancy caused the damage (Fig. 7.1).

Further research learned that the teratogenic effect only occurred in some animal species. It was found that in some rabbit species the effect was seen when the compound was administered between the eighth and sixteenth day of pregnancy whereas mice did not show this effect at all.

This thalidomide tragedy led to the US Kefauver Harris Amendment or "Drug Efficacy Amendment" which is a 1962 amendment to the Federal

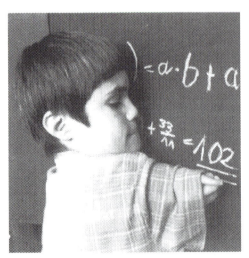

FIGURE 7.1   Photo of child with phocomelia. *The image used from "The Horror and Hope of Thalidomide." As published in www.chm.bris.ac.uk/motm/thalidomide/effects.html.*

Food, Drug, and Cosmetic Act. From that time onward, drug manufacturers were required to provide proof of the effectiveness *and* safety of drugs before approval. Also in Europe, the first European pharmaceutical directive (Directive 65/65/EEC, which dates from January 1965) was a reaction to the thalidomide tragedy and harmonized standards for authorization on approval of proprietary medicinal products. Teratogenic potential of a new drug was from that time on tested in at least three different animal species.

In this way was the toxicological finding leading in defining regulation. Sadly, some years ago the toxicity of thalidomide in babies was observed again in Brazil. In this case the "miracle drug" was administered to elderly woman to treat their leprosy. It appeared to be effective and the mothers conveniently passed the drug on to their daughters. Unaware of the dangers, pregnancy in some instances tragically resulted in phocomelia.

Interestingly, the drug has recently found new applications in the lung disease sarcoidosis and also in the treatment of cancer where it inhibits the sprouting of blood vessels (the angiogenesis) in the solid tumor. The severity of the problem warranted and in fact received political and regulatory actions.

However, even after these regulations, new problems arose indicating the necessity to be really cautious in administering drugs to pregnant women. Diethylstilbesterol (DES) is a synthetic nonsteroidal estrogen which was prescribed to women who has one or more miscarriages hoping to prevent those miscarriages. Although the effect was very doubtful, physicians remained prescribing DES until at least 1971. At that time it was recognized that in utero DES exposure of daughters of women who took the drug had a high chance of developing cancer of the vagina and cervix.

In 1971 the US Food and Drug Administration made a public warning on the use of DES by pregnant women. Unfortunately various countries in Europe continued the use of DES until the early 1980s. The DES daughters acquired more problems, like distortions of the uterus, lack of fertility, more vaginal discharge, and delivering more breech babies. The DES mothers between the age of 45 and 65 had a higher chance of breast cancer. In the Netherlands for example it was prescribed between 1947 and even until 1976. Amazing and regrettable that it took so long before the evident toxicological warnings were taken seriously. Learning of mistakes remains difficult.

What certainly remains is deep caution with regard to prescribing drugs to pregnant woman. It is also realized that many dietary ingredients are not safe for pregnant woman (Fig. 7.2).

FROM LEGISLATION TO TOXICOLOGY

More frequently, the reverse occurs, namely legislation dictates the toxicological approach that should be used. A recent example is the novel foods legislation. In many countries around the world, guidance documents have been published on the safety assessment on novel foods. A novel food should

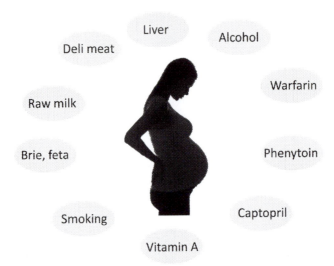

FIGURE 7.2 List of food, food derived ingredients, and drugs not safe for pregnant women.

be safe to consume and well labeled not to mislead consumers. The traditional approach for compounds is setting an acceptable daily intake (ADI) that entails a 100-fold safety margin when compared with the lowest no observable adverse effect level (NOAEL) in animals. This routine is not feasible for most novel foods which are complex in nature (Chapter 5: From Prevention to Precaution—Valuing Risks).

In the European Union it has been attempted to harmonize the authorization and use of novel foods and food ingredients since 1997 when the Regulation (EC) No. 258/97 on novel food and novel food ingredients was adopted. Novel food is defined as any food not consumed by humans within the European Union to a significant degree prior to May 15, 1997. It can be food with a new intentionally modified molecular structure. Food consisting of, isolated from, or produced from microorganisms, fungi, or algae, or from material of mineral origin, or food from cell culture or tissue, culture from animals or plants, and so on.

The regulation was further amended and lastly in 2015 in Regulation (EU) No. 2015/2283. The regulation will come into effect in January 2018. The European Food Safety Authority (EFSA) involved the various stakeholders via public consultation in finalizing the guidance documents. Quite some information has to be delivered (Fig. 7.3).

Besides information on the biological source, quantitative and qualitative data on the composition and possible impurities should also be provided. Hazards that may arise during packaging or storage should be identified. Proposed use and anticipated intake should be described. The toxicological information that should be provided includes a battery of in vitro tests to

11.12.2015   EN   Official Journal of the European Union   L 327/1

REGULATION (EU) 2015/2283 OF THE EUROPEAN PARLIAMENT AND OF THE COUNCIL

of 25 November 2015

on novel foods, amending Regulation (EU) No 1169/2011 of the European Parliament and of the Council and repealing Regulation (EC) No 258/97 of the European Parliament and of the Council and Commission Regulation (EC) No 1852/2001

FIGURE 7.3   Front page of the Novel Food Regulation.

check for genotoxicity. In case of a positive result, in vivo studies should follow, e.g., a 90-day repeated dose toxicity study checking for neurotoxic, immunological, reproductive organ, or endocrine-mediated effects. The outcome of this subchronic toxicity study might form the trigger for a chronic toxicity or carcinogenicity study. In human toxicity studies, physical examination, studies on blood chemistry, urine analysis, blood pressure, and organ function tests may follow. In case the novel food exerts the so-called pharmacodynamics effects, specific studies may be required to ensure the novel food does not raise any safety concerns.

Explanations about the Novel Regulation in guidance documents describe simple and rather outdated toxicological methodology to ensure the safety. Novel techniques and notions about toxicology are not suggested. Why is the regulatory authority old-fashioned? Does it offer more security? Is the Novel Food regulation necessary because an immense toxicological problem exists or does it sprout from a general public sense of danger? Does society demand an extensive safety regulation? Obviously, our reflections on precautionary culture do give some pointers to answer such questions.

SOME TOXIC LIMITS SEEM TO BE CARVED IN STONE

Once limits of some sort have been established, it seems that these values sometimes firmly remain set and cannot be modified easily. New convincing knowledge will not always readily lead to change of threshold concentrations. An interesting example is nitrate.

Nitrate in drinking water has for decades been thought to be the cause of which is called the "blue baby syndrome," infantile methemoglobinemia. Nitrate changes the hemoglobin (the transporter of oxygen in the red blood cells) via the reduced form of nitrate, nitrite, into methemoglobin, a state of hemoglobin in which the iron is oxidized and is in the Fe^{3+} form which is unable to deliver oxygen to tissues. Transport of oxygen becomes hampered and a shortage of oxygen, cyanosis, leads to the bluish color of the intoxicated young child.

This general belief was fueled by the notion that infants under 6 months of age have a higher vulnerability for methemoglobin compared to adults because of lower enzyme activity to reduce the methemoglobin thus restoring the oxygen transport in the first months of life. Because victims of methemoglobinemia showed to have drunk nitrate containing well water, nitrate was blamed for this effect. Moreover it was known that nitrite is more toxic for hemoglobin than nitrate and even children that did not drink nitrate contaminated water belonged to the victims.

That led to the suggestion that a bacterial infection in the gastrointestinal tract might be involved in the conversion of nitrate to nitrite, which was the ultimate cause of the toxicity. It led to a strict regulation for nitrate in drinking water. The World Health Organization (WHO) established a maximum level of 50 mg/L of nitrate in drinking water. This had huge consequences in rural areas where nitrate in soil water exists as a consequence of the use of nitrate containing fertilizers. A stream of reports followed indicating that even infants, without exposure to high-nitrate drinking water but with symptoms of diarrhea, could suffer from methemoglobinemia. Suggestions to reexamine the strict WHO maximum levels because diarrhea appeared a causative role in methemoglobinemia were largely neglected.

It was subsequently found that in response to colonic inflammation several tissues produced nitric oxide (NO) via an enzyme called nitric oxide synthase. The NO oxidizes to nitrite and nitrate. Endogenously formed NO may thus eventually result in the methemoglobinemia observed in young children as a result of drinking bacterial contaminated water. It was for a long time thought that it was the combination of bacterial contamination and nitrate which could lead to methemoglobinemia.

Despite persistent regulatory and scientific focus on the risks of exposure to nitrate, new scientific perspectives emerged once NO was discovered to be a major physiological chemical component. This discovery created a multifaceted image on the role of nitrate, but also nitrite, in human physiology. NO production has been shown to be vital to maintain normal blood circulation and defense against infection. NO, subsequently, is oxidized via nitrite to nitrate, which is conserved by the kidneys and concentrated in the saliva. The discovery of NO as a vital physiological chemical explains the common knowledge that mammals produce nitrate de novo. Mayerhofer already observed this as early as 1913. Infections yield the most noticeable instance of nitrate biosynthesis, explaining methemoglobinemia as a result of intestinal infections that reduce nitrate to the deleterious nitrite, and not exposure to exogenous nitrate as such.

It is now recognized that nitrate may even have beneficial effects because it can be reduced (e.g., by mouth and intestinal bacteria) into NO which may lead to decrease in blood pressure. Nitrate-rich vegetables may thus have a beneficial effect on blood pressure. It is amazing how a compound-like nitrate changes its face from extremely toxic to health promoting. The health limits, though, remain the same, indeed carved in stone it seems. Apparently it is very difficult to change existing views based on new facts about certain chemical compounds such as nitrate.

WHAT DETERMINES THE CHOICE OF TOPICS FOR TOXICOLOGICAL REGULATIONS?

A major determinant leading for human behavior is fear. Plain fear. Fear is an important regulator of our peripheral autonomic nervous system. The autonomic nervous system controls the function of our internal organs and acts largely unconsciously on for example the heart, respiration, and digestion. The autonomic nervous system can be divided into two branches—the sympathetic and the parasympathetic nervous system. The sympathetic branch is accountable for the flight—fright—fight response, while the parasympathetic nervous system is regarded as the rest—digest responsible branch. The nerves involved in the rapid excitatory sympathetic system are intensely interconnected which leads to a rapid overwhelming primary flight—fright—fight response. This response has to be quick because survival depends on it.

Fear elicits this response, action is needed, and a thoughtless reflex response is provoked. Fear is a main human driver and it is easy to envision that perceived toxicity leads to sympathetic preparedness to request toxicological regulation. This is very much in line with precautionary culture we discussed earlier. Indeed, historian Joanna Bourke observed: "fear of crime was not the most potent dogging late 20th century societies. There was another category of danger that frightened many Britons and Americans as the century staggered to its conclusion: ecological degradation." Part of that ecological degradation is deemed to be related to industrially produced synthetic chemicals.

Another factor that stimulates the quest for politicians and regulators to react on sometimes relatively small toxicological problems is the currently rapid communication. Small accidents are enlarged by the rapid communication. An occurrence in a distant location in the world is news within minutes. The consumer receives all kinds of information rapidly from different channels and asks for action.

Moreover, messages on toxicities keep on circulating. The proverbial "tomorrow's fish which is wrapped up in today's newspaper" is not valid anymore. Bad news, and unfortunately most news is bad, remains visible on the World Wide Web. It will further enlarge toxicologically cultured mishaps.

The feeling that (putative) large calamities are not dealt with properly by the authorities will easily give rise to conspiracy theories. Food scares are blown up to astronomical proportions and the emotion that responsible authorities do not act appropriately persists.

Contradictory, the fact that all the information is available nowadays generates the situation that only a small part of it can actually be read. It is just impossible to read the vast pile of literature (see also Chapter 8: Knowledge vs Insight). The consequence is that a selection is made of the all blogs, vlogs, articles, etc., someone will see and read. This selection is easily made within one's framework: those outings that are pleasing to the reader, i.e., notions that fit in one's own line of thinking will preferably be absorbed.

This is also known as confirmation bias. Concepts and views that are not in harmony with one's belief can easily be disregarded.

Other confirmation biases are formed by search engines like Google or Yahoo. Once you requested information on a certain toxicological problem, Google provides you with suggestions for novel selections along the same lines. In this way the natural propensity to most value information that confirms own ideas becomes reinforced. It becomes increasingly difficult to objectively obtain insights, which enable well-balanced legislative structures. Thus, legislation and regulation that leave enough freedom to research and innovation but at the same time fill in the gaps is needed. How do we protect the patient from cognitive impairment that may occur from polypharmacy (*vide supra*)?

REFERENCES AND FURTHER READING

Bates, R., 1999. What Risk? Butterworth-Heinemann, Oxford.

Blaauboer, B.J., Boobis, A.R., Bradford, B., Cockburn, A., Constable, A., Daneshian, M., et al., 2016. Considering new methodologies in strategies for safety assessment of foods and food ingredients. Food Chem. Toxicol. 91, 19−35.

Bourke, J., 2005. Fear. A Cultural History. Virago Press, London, UK.

Catel, W., Tunger, H., 1933. Über das Vorkommen von Nitrate (und Nitrit) im Harn junger Saülinge bei ausschliesslicher Frauenmilchernährung. Jahrbuch für Kinderheilkunde 140, 253−262.

Furchgott, R.F., Zawadzki, J.V., 1980. The obligatory role of endothelial cells in the relaxation of arterial smooth muscle by acetylcholine. Nature. 288, 373−376.

Hanekamp, J.C., Bast, A., Kwakman, J.H., 2012. Of reductionism and the pendulum swing: connecting toxicology and human health. Dose Response 10 (2), 155−176.

< http://ec.europa.eu/food/safety/novel_food/legislation_en > (accessed 12.01.17).

< http://www.agingbraincare.org/tools/abc-anticholinergic-cognitive-burden-scale/ >

< http://www.agingbraincare.org/uploads/products/ACB_scale_-_legal_size.pdf > (12.01.17).

Lundberg, J.O., Weitzberg, E., Gladwin, M.T., 2008. The nitrate−nitrite−nitric oxide pathway in physiology and therapeutics. Nature Rev. Drug Disc. 7 (2), 156−167.

Mayerhofer, E., 1913. Der Harn des Saülings Ergebnisse der inneren. Medizin und Kinderheilkunde 12, 553−618.

Moncada, S.M., Palmer, R.M.J., Higgs, E.A., 1991. Nitric oxide: physiology, pathophysiology, and pharmacology. Pharmacol. Rev. 43, 109−142.

Nilsson, R., Sjöström, H., 1972. Thalidomide and the power of the drug companies (a Penguin special). Penguin Books Ltd, Middlesex, England.

Schrager, S., Potter, B.E., 2004. Diethylstilbesterol (DES) exposure. Am. Fam. Physician. 69, 2395−2400.

Vrolijk, M.F., Opperhuizen, A., Jansen, E.H., Bast, A., Haenen, G.R., 2015. Anticholinergic accumulation: a slumbering interaction between drugs and food supplements. Basic Clin. Pharmacol. Toxicol. 117 (6), 427−432.

Weseler, A.R., Bast, A., 2010. Oxidative stress and vascular function: implications for pharmacologic treatment. Curr. Hypertens. Rep. 12, 154−161.

Chapter 8

Knowledge vs Insight

Michael Polanyi was one of the world's leading physical chemists in the first half of the 20th century, and a leading philosopher of science in the second half of that same century. His experimental and theoretical work on gas adsorption by solids (activated carbon to begin with), on which he first published during the Great War (1914–18), is still being referred to and used to this very day. The Polanyi theory has been recognized as one of the most powerful theories for dealing with both gas and aqueous adsorption on heterogeneous solid surfaces. In his defense of his specific theory of adsorption in the first decades of the 20th century, however, the mainstream scientific community rejected his ideas in favor of the work done by Langmuir, despite the fact that his theory carried strong experimental papers. That changed in the 1950s and 1960s. Interestingly, while reflecting, as a philosopher of science, on his initial failure to convince the scientific community of his approach, he stated in his 1963 *Science* article that "at all times [there must be] a predominantly accepted scientific view of the nature of things, in the light of which research is jointly conducted by members of the community of scientists. A strong presumption that any evidence which contradicts this view is invalid must prevail. ... The dangers of suppressing or disregarding evidence that runs counter to orthodox views about the nature of things are, of course, notorious, and they have often proved disastrous. Science guards against these dangers, up to a point, by allowing some measure of dissent from its orthodoxy. But scientific opinion has to consider and decide, at its own ultimate risk, how far it can allow such tolerance to go, if it is not to admit for publication so much nonsense that scientific journals are rendered worthless thereby." Within this age of informatics available to all, yet not always easy to get to grips with by specialists and nonspecialists alike, Polanyi gives us ample material to reflect upon. Here, we will try to order some of the issues the field of toxicology is confronted with.

THE WORLD AT LARGE

As we have shown in the previous pages, chemistry is everywhere. And it has a myriad of effects on us in untold ways. In toxicology we try to fathom these exposures and effects. For that, many different research fields are tapped into from chemistry to biology, from pharmacology to medicine, and

Toxicology: What Everyone Should Know. DOI: http://dx.doi.org/10.1016/B978-0-12-805348-5.00008-9

also from food science to healthy diets and from toxicology to hazard identification and risk regulation, etc.

Clearly, the identification of hazards of chemicals, as discussed earlier, seems to be of prime importance in our precautionary culture. Risks of chemicals exposure of especially the man-made kind need to be banished as much as possible: better safe than sorry. That has, to some extent, driven the growth of scientific research into the risks of modernity, in which chemical risks play a notable part.

Subsequently, thousands of scientist toxicologists publish their findings in many different peer-reviewed journals. Their scientific careers, in large part, are built thereon. Better, these findings need to be made available through the media to the general public as to make one's research more relevant. Once talked about in the press, academic standing increases and thereby the chance to get grant proposals accepted.

It should not be surprising that the theme of risk plays a prominent role in these public outings. Nowadays, many different risk issues take front page: killer asteroids, global influenza, fertility risks because of pesticides on our veggies, and so on. We are continually warned that, for the human race, "time is running out" unless we do something about global warming or climate change. "The end is nigh" is no longer a warning issued by the religiously inclined, far from it. In fact, scaremongering is increasingly represented as an act of concerned and responsible citizenship. And scientists are among those responsible citizens.

But there are problems. To begin with, the number of specialized academic journals and published articles is such that it is impossible for anyone to keep track of, including the academic specialist. Moreover, it seems that only a handful of people, usually colleagues, will ever read those individual articles. Even fewer articles will ever make it to the general public through the many different media outlets—national and local newspapers, magazines, news websites, blogs, vlogs, and so on. And that fact alone does not carry any seal of quality. Indeed, the bias toward risk is well understood by many as a means to come into the spotlights of public attention. So-called "fake news" is the talk of the town and how to identify it as such is no easy task.

All sorts of (selected) information are available to almost all, yet weighing its relevance is far more difficult. Additionally, in what ways are the topics that toxicological research focuses on governed: by regulatory agencies, media, fear (see the previous chapter), politics, public awareness, or internal academic drivers such as curiosity, professional responsibility? Are hazards and risks the main drivers therein? And how do we sift through the available material and make coherent sense of it all?

An analogy with the definition of health we defend in this book seems to be applicable here. If the ability to adapt is the defining character of human health on the biological level, then the ability to keep one's mental health should be driven by a "reasonable" homeostasis with the outside world of (dis)information to which we are exposed. That, however, requires some

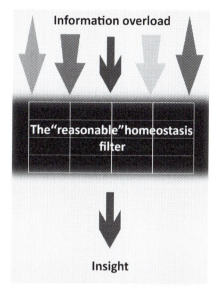

FIGURE 8.1 Picture of information overload and the "reasonable" homeostasis filter (see further below).

kind of "mental mechanism": discarding the junk and keeping the good stuff as not to poison ourselves with disinformation (Fig. 8.1).

Such a mental mechanism should be available not only to the specialist but to everyone. We will propose three insights from the philosophy of science and will subsequently rework them into some straightforward "tools" and apply these to a few examples from the realm of toxicology that reached the spotlights of public and political attention.

Overall, we should be wary of the law of inverse rationality. We can be sensibly rational at the fringe of our interests, where the prospect for prideful self-assertion is limited. Conversely, when a certain topic approaches the core of our being—our wealth, health, safety, security, and longevity—the greater the probability, that truth will be subsidiary to other values (e.g., human autonomy, self-preservation, fear, power). We will explore this further in the following section.

OF SCIENCE AND THE WORLD—THREE INSIGHTS

It might seem that we have wandered into the field of neuroscience and related topics in order to understand the "mechanism for mental health," if we could identify some such. That is not the case. What we do here is formulating a few notions—insights—that could be a means to evaluate scientific statements that capture the imagination of the press, the public, policymakers, and the like. These insights are derived from the philosophy of science. *They invite to be attentive, intelligent, critical, and responsible.*

The corollaries of the insights will be subsequently expressed in some tools. These could help the nonspecialist through the endless news items and policy prescriptions related to the benefits of certain foods or food supplements, the purported dangers of rubber granulate-containing artificial turf to young soccer players, the risks of sunlight in general and sunbathing in particular, the occurrence of child leukemia ostensibly induced by nonionizing electromagnetic fields, say, from overhead power lines, and so on.

Science is usually understood as empirical in nature (although mathematics and (scientific) reasoning cannot be reduced thereto). Through experimentation one tries to establish basic regularities of the world (Fig 8.2). What the empirical sciences produce are *contingent* propositions, that is *not necessarily* true or false: "chemical A interacts with protein X resulting in effect Y"; "the element thallium has the atomic weight of 204.38"; "the lethal dose of X for mice is Y"; "the consumption of this food adds to our health and longevity".

These and many other propositions generated by the empirical sciences are all *conditionally* true, given various facts and evidence. None of these propositions are logically necessary. It is logically possible for these statements to be false, say, due to measurement errors, mistakes in experimental setups, incorrect starting materials, the limitations of available facts, and so on. Thus, scientific arguments start from empirical premises and draw only probabilistic conclusions, prone to correction. To be sure, we do not doubt

GREAT EVENTS IN CHEMISTRY

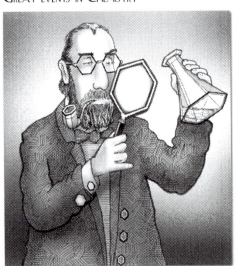

1865: Kekulé, moments before his brilliant insight into the structure of benzene.

FIGURE 8.2 Friedrich August Kekulé moments before "discovering" benzene (Nick D. Kim http://scienceandink.com/).

the measurements of the atomic weight of thallium, for instance. The premise of trust is ever present, and quite rightly so. But, as the business of science expands, this premise is undermined, as we will see.

Here, the *first* insight emerges: no scientific results will give us *definitive* answers to our many questions. Many scientists, perhaps following too closely the citizen or policy cheering section, developed the risky habit of insisting that their *conditional* truths are *necessary* truths. Some have gone further downhill by insisting fallaciously that their probable truths are universally true. The compelling statement "science has shown that . . ." should be taken with a grain of salt, and sometimes perhaps even more than that, say, a truckload. Wholesome skepticism thus is a balancing act, as Polanyi showed, between orthodoxy and dissent, between the quietist "everybody knows that . . ." and the twitchy "forget everything you know about . . .".

To be sure, ignoring counterevidence in order to maintain the theory under investigation is not uncommon among scientists, and that may be the right way to respond. This is not just a rationally informed decision. The passionate commitment informs the scientist to stick to his guns. The institution of science could hardly survive if all or most members made it their aim to falsify theories in the sense of trying to generate anomalies. Progress in science requires that most scientists get themselves in the grip of a theory which they aim to develop and defend it, without simply trying to dispose of it as quickly as possible. This might equally result in the scientist overshooting the mark in order to avoid professional embarrassment when he persists with an increasingly unmaintainable theory.

The *second* insight, incipient in this debate on (the limits of) commitment, seems, at first glance, to conflict with the first one. That, however, is unwarranted. There is much more to scientific results than merely some viewpoints expressed by experts. We *can* and *do* have a sense of understanding of the world that exists independently of our current knowledge.

But, that requires that we steer well clear of two notions that undermine any attempt to try to come to such growing understanding. One is the false belief that "everything is an opinion" whereby all utterances of human understanding are no more than personal edicts that by definition cannot be contested. After all, here there is no frame of reference that surpasses the personal. The other is the equally false belief that human inquiry can become all-encompassing explicitly with the aid of science. This is also known as *scientism*: that is the fallacious idea that only one type of human understanding—science—is in control of the entire universe *and* what can be said about it (Fig. 8.3).

The philosopher Thomas Nagel gave fair warning about our understanding of the world around us that captures both contradictory aspects of our culture that seem so far apart yet are so closely intertwined: ". . . for objectivity is both underrated and overrated, sometimes by the same persons. It is underrated by those who don't regard it as a method of understanding the world as it is in itself. It is overrated by those who believe it can provide a complete view of the world on its own, replacing the subjective views from

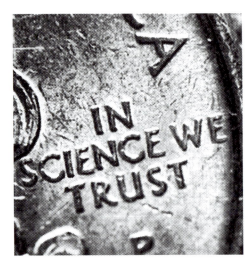

FIGURE 8.3   In science we trust.

which it has developed. These errors are connected: they both stem from an insufficiently robust sense of reality and of its independence of any particular form of human understanding."

The term "objectivity" involves some kind of impartiality, a lack of bias, basically distinguishing between two ways of forming beliefs about the hidden structure of the world. One way depends on, say, caprice, prejudice, expectations, power, pride, wealth, fear, etc., the lower nonepistemic interests, and drivers that are *unrelated* to genuine knowledge gathering. The other avoids such inacceptable influences. But just avoiding these pitfalls simply won't do.

Doing proper science involves robust ethical and fiduciary-type commitments: there is no discovery in science without the passionate aspiration *to know*, and a belief (as in trust) that there is something out there *to know*. Passion, love, and faith (again, as in trust) sustain the method of science *a priori*, providing for the higher interests (in contrast to the lower ones stated previously) scientists need to embrace to actually become good scientists. Clinical cold-eyed realism demands all manner of epistemic virtues, that is related to the gathering of knowledge: openness to being wrong, selflessness, humility, generosity of spirit, hard labor, curiosity, tenacity, a readiness to collaborate, conscientious judgment, transparency, and the like. For the famous philosopher Thomas Aquinas, all such virtues have their source in love. Love is the ultimate form of undeceived realism. That is why it is intimately related to truth (Fig. 8.4).

This brings us to the *third* insight. A scientist faithful to the scientific ideals of judiciousness and honest self-criticism will present her or his results with humility and an acute awareness that the world out there is much bigger than the results presented. Drawing conclusions that go far beyond the published work is a sure sign of an overestimation of what can actually be said.

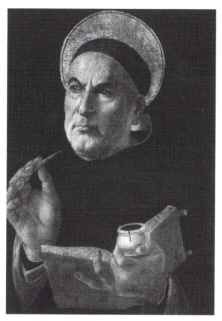

FIGURE 8.4   Thomas Aquinas by Sandro Botticelli. *From Granger—Historical Picture Archive.*

The context within which the presented work figures is essential, and without it judging the quality of the published material, even superficially, is almost impossible to do. Cherry picking (also known as the exception fallacy), that is basing general conclusions on a minor subset of cases, is a real-world problem and a big one to boot.

These three insights give leeway to a number of "tools" that could add to a general understanding of scientific information that finds its way to mainstream media and Internet websites everywhere. Lest we forget, both institutionally and personally, science is looked at as a discerning field of advice in terms of numerous aspects of life, such as geographical position and direction (think of the Global Positioning System), human health (medicine, food security and safety, nutrition and health, particulate matter air pollution, cell phone radiation, etc.), parenthood (the "nanny shows" with its pedagogical experts once were broadcasting blockbusters). We increasingly believe that experts can inform us reliably and definitively about the status of the world with respect to many central characteristics of our personal and corporate lives. And the idea that that is compulsory is typical for precautionary culture we discussed in Chapter 5, From Prevention to Precaution—Valuing Risks.

THE "REASONABLE" HOMEOSTASIS—SOME EXEMPLIFIED TOOLS

Thus, the scientific endeavor, however incomplete, is focused on probing the hidden structure of reality—of atoms and molecules, of proteins and organs, of neurology and psychology, of social relations and politics, and so on. Results, which give insight into the world we live in, are nevertheless conditional and always open to extension or even partial or complete revision. If scientists are to be successful in delivering insights with proper objectivity and humility, then our knowledge base will grow steadily, with its backwards and forwards included.

However, the precautionary drive toward (scientific) surety about the world and us—related to our safety, security, health, and longevity—embeds a number of shortcomings into the scientific institution that surface once the three insights mentioned are confronted with this drive. Here, a few tools, based in part on the work done by Ioannidis, are presented to appraise claims made by the scientific community, while not being a specialist. We deliberately state the tools in the negative form as a device to reverse the seriousness with which scientific results are sometimes presented. These tools should not be understood as directly causal: "if ..., then ...". Rather, they are indicators to make nonspecialists aware and critical of the research results presented. The question "But is it true?" should always be in the back of one's mind, whether a specialist or not.

1. *The smaller the effect sizes in any scientific field, the less likely the research findings are true (insights 1, 2, and 3).*

Scientists are increasingly obliged to target smaller effect sizes purportedly related to everyday agents to which we are exposed. Usually, the potential effects of certain agents are theoretical: they are derived from models without actually observing those effects in human populations. In fact, such observation is impossible as any effect, if at all existent, is simply far too small to actually measure. Think for instance of the proverbial singular carcinogenic molecule, as discussed in Chapter 6, Molecular Trepidations—The Linear Nonthreshold Model, being able to cause cancer in an individual after exposure.

The result is, so the story goes, insight into how we can protect ourselves from even the most mundane risks. This has been called the "epidemic of apprehension." And this epidemic grows with each new alarm about a new "menace in daily life." Although this notion was first put forward by Alvan Feinstein some three decades ago, this purported menace has grown, aided by our precautionary propensities.

The exposure to radon—a radioactive noble gas that is exuded by natural stony materials such as granite but also building materials—and the prevalence of lung cancer are examples here. In 1999, considering the approximately 157,000 lung cancer deaths occurring annually in the United States, radon was *computed* to play a role in about 15,000–22,000 cases.

In 2005, many news outlets in the Netherlands reported that particulate matter (PM) air pollution resulted in 18,000 deaths per year. This number was based on reports of the Dutch Environment and Nature Planning Bureau and the National Institute for Public Health and

Environmental Hygiene. Again, this worrying figure was the result of models computations. Below we will reflect on these numbers further.

2. *The more fashionable a scientific field is (with more scientific teams involved in the research area), the less likely the research findings are true (insight 3).*

Science, as any other human endeavor, has its fads. With numerous research teams working on the same issues in a certain field and with immense experimental data being generated, timing is of the essence in defeating the competition. Thus, each team may prioritize on pursuing and disseminating its most impressive "positive" results.

"Negative" results may become attractive for dissemination if some other team has found a "positive" association on the same question first. In that case, it may be attractive to refute a claim made in some respected journal. Consequently, rapidly alternating extreme research claims and markedly opposite refutations is indicative of this state of affairs, which is of great interest to the media as well. When such alternating extreme opposites of results and views from the scientific community are presented in the media, chances are that neither have any truth in them.

3. *The greater the the probability of the presence of nonobjective lower interests—caprice, prejudice, expectations, power, pride, wealth, fear—in a scientific field, the less likely the research findings are true (insight 3).*

When opportunities to gather large sums of money are available within a certain academic field, the quality of research findings is bound to drop. Usually this is understood within commercial settings. Yet, the same holds true for research done by means of public funding.

What often is forgotten is that governments have vested interests to push certain political agendas bolstered with scientific findings. Think for instance of the European REACH regulation (Registration, Evaluation, Authorization and Restriction of Chemicals). For more than a 100,000 chemicals, biological, chemical, physical, and toxicological data needs to be gathered and reported as a means to protect human health and the environment from the risks that can be posed by chemicals.

We do not say anything new that chemophobia (prejudice, power, fear) is one of the nonepistemic drivers of REACH, as is made clear in the precursory "Strategy for a future Chemicals Policy" whitepaper of the European Commission in 2001 in which the "protection of human health and promotion of a nontoxic environment" is one of the key elements of REACH. As we have already seen, there is no such thing as a "nontoxic environment". Indeed, it is an incomprehensible term not conducive for life on earth, including our own.

Incidentally, we should be wary of the genetic fallacy. This fallacy is committed when a proposition is accepted or rejected because of its origin, history, who speaks it, or who paid for it to be spoken. This fallacy is nothing other than an irregular and remote proxy of the actual content of the proposition. The latter should always be assessed on its own merits, and nothing else.

4. *The more reductionist and consensus-driven a scientific field is, the less likely the research findings are true (insight 1).*

When scientists within an academic field press for consensus around a certain cherished hypothesis, chances are that they try to block competing and tenable hypotheses for reasons other than the higher scientific interests. Consequently, chances are that research findings are less likely to be true. If the consensus hypothesis is strongly reductionist, whereby the scientistic fallacy looms large, things are aggravated. Although ignoring counterevidence in order to maintain the hypothesis under investigation is common, *forcing* consensus seems eccentric in the light of the well-documented fallibility of scientific understanding.

The late 19th-century luminiferous ether that postulated a medium (the ether) for the propagation of light is perhaps the most *famous* example of a generally accepted yet false scientific theory. It was invoked to explicate the ability of the wave-based light to propagate through empty (vacuous) space; something that waves should not be able to do. The most *infamous* scientific theory that was abandoned *and* repudiated is undoubtedly eugenics ("good origin"). This was the "science" of applying principles of genetics and heredity for the purpose of "improving" the human race and was a "settled science" by the end of the 19th century. It was seen as necessary for the preservation of society (Fig. 8.5).

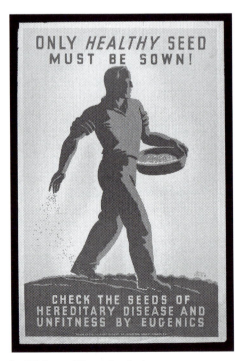

FIGURE 8.5 Eugenics (Wellcome Library, London).

Investigators may suppress, for instance via the peer review process, the appearance and dissemination of findings that refute their own findings, perpetuating in their fields outdated or even false hypotheses and theories. The ousting of legitimate research that voice dissenting views is indicative of the fact that the truth content of research findings is under pressure.

Previously, we have discussed the linear nonthreshold (LNT) model and its faults, which are manifold. The consensus view in favor of the LNT still holds but it seems that more empirical views of dose−responses are finding their way in research and policy. Low and high doses differ in the responses they generate and are not linearly related by default. Assessing the extremes of exposure to generate the majority of the effects of exposure is the unnoticed fallacy the LNT harbors.

Reviewing all this, what are we to say about the menace in daily life and the ways in which this is researched and communicated? Some exposure to some substance might be said to "double the risk." But, if the *actual* risk goes from one in a billion to two in a billion, you only have an actual risk of two in a billion. Which is completely trivial. So, the *context* of actual risk— the doubling of one to two in a billion—is crucial in understanding what's going on. Rarely is such a context given.

Another issue is *practical* risk. If you have a high *actual* risk that only applies to a few people, the practical risk for the total population is still quite small. An extreme example will illustrate this: a risk of one in a million for 99 people (not exposed) is compared to a risk of 10 in a million for one person (exposed). We are talking here of a 10-fold increase in risk! Which sounds scary, no doubt. But the actual risk is still small for the total population of all 100 people within a population of a million.

A saner and less hyperbolic practice of science, one that is not quite so dictatorial and inflexible, one that is calmer and in less of a hurry, one that is far less sure of itself, one that has a proper appreciation of how much it doesn't know would benefit specialist and nonspecialist alike. However, there is much deserved and legitimate angst about the "reproducibility crisis" which afflicts those fields which (over-)rely on statistical methods. For instance, how do scientists tease out ever-smaller agent effects on our health as discussed in tool number 1? And is there any way to reproduce these results?

Actually, as we already discussed, observation is impossible here as any effect, if at all existent, is simply far too small to measure. Usually probabilistic (statistical) models play the dominant role. Probabilistic models are not causal, and can never lead to certainty. Probabilities (What are the chances that …?) are stand-ins for knowledge of causes; consequently these probabilities do not become and can never be causes themselves.

Nevertheless, these models are presented as to produce real-world public health information: 18,000 deaths because of PM air pollution in the Netherlands; 15,000−22,000 radon-related lung cancer deaths in the United

States. This in fact is the iniquity of reification, as we have seen before. This happens when models are regarded as real-world creatures. They are not. Reification happens, far too often, when we fail to recall that our mathematical creations are abstractions and not reality. And that rules out proper reproduction as real-world checks and balances are missing (Fig. 8.6).

One important reason why it is often thought probability models can discern cause is because of hidden bias. The bias is uncovered by thinking about who decides what goes into the databases as potential causes or proxies of causes. As Briggs explains: "Consider the proposition 'Bob spent $1124.52 on his credit card.' This 'effect' might have been caused by the sock colors of the residents of Perth, say, or the number of sucker sticks longer than 3 inches in the town of Gaylord, Michigan, or anything. These odd possibilities are not in databases of credit card charges, because database creators cannot imagine how these oddities are in any way causative of the effect of interest. Items which 'make the cut' are there because creators can imagine how these items are causes, or how they might facilitate or block other causes, and this is because the natures or essences of these items are known to some extent. ..." Consequently, the results are no more than the biases of the researchers they infused in their model *a priori*.

Another major issue is "control." Tributary "variables" are entered into models and are said to be "controls" like age, gender, weight, smoking, alcohol use, genetics, and so on. The attempt here is that the agent under scrutiny and its effects are "isolated" from all sorts of other agents

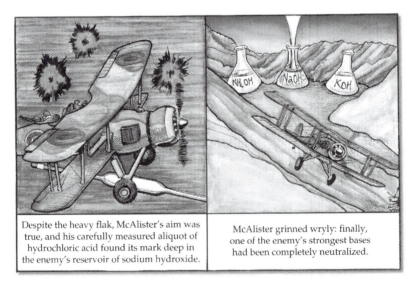

Despite the heavy flak, McAlister's aim was true, and his carefully measured aliquot of hydrochloric acid found its mark deep in the enemy's reservoir of sodium hydroxide.

McAlister grinned wryly: finally, one of the enemy's strongest bases had been completely neutralized.

FIGURE 8.6 Reification cartoon (Nick D. Kim http://scienceandink.com/).

that might have similar effects as the one studied. The word "control" here is deceiving, and in fact a gross misnomer. Despite the many "controls" that can be infused into the model, there will always be other characteristics that are not or cannot be controlled for, because for instance they are unknown. The term "control" thus is the complete opposite of the truth of the matter.

Moreover, "controls" are usually (rough) proxies of actual causes. Take for instance gender. In athletic sports such as the 100 m, men gold medalists are faster than the fastest women. Does male sex as such cause the men to outrace feminine competitors? Far from it; gender does not determine that at all. Instead, gender causes differences in anatomy and physiology that are tied to differing athletic performance.

This is why the countless models that "control" for gender and which imply gender is "a cause" are always wrong (unless they are modeling direct effects of sex, such as pregnancy, and in which case, no model is used because we understand the essence). Gender is a proxy for (usually) multiple other causes and is itself not a cause. And this kind of reasoning also applies for things such as race, income, and education. Statistical models simply aren't capable of discerning cause.

So, is there any moral to the story of science, models, knowledge, and insights. We think there is. Perhaps the most important one is that any theory or model in science should be verified by making *predictions of observables* never (*as in never*) seen before. A good scientist, aware of at least the three (much repeated and straightforward) insights we have posited in this chapter, asks the pertinent questions, designs the experiments, collects the data in a transparent and accessible manner, builds the model, and then, every single time, this model must be used to make predictions. As the Dilbert-cartoonist Scott Adams proposed in his blog of the December 28, 2016 (much to the chagrin of a quite a few commentators):

> So today's challenge is to find a working scientist or PhD in some climate-related field who will agree with the idea that the climate science models do a good job of predicting the future. ... Remind your scientist that as far as you know there has never been a multi-year, multi-variable, complicated model of any type that predicted anything with useful accuracy. Case in point: The experts and their models said Trump had no realistic chance of winning.
>
> Your scientist will fight like a cornered animal to conflate the credibility of the measurements and the basic science of CO_2 with the credibility of the pro-jection models. Don't let that happen. Make your scientist tell you that compli-cated multi-variable projections models that span years are credible. Or not.

This will help further the practice of science that is, more precisely should be, judicious and honestly self-critical. And it will help the citizens of this world. If predictions of certain pet theories of scientists go awry on an almost daily basis, forget about it. It's just fake news.

REFERENCES AND FURTHER READING

Adams, S. *The Climate Science Challenge*. December 28, 2016. See <http://blog.dilbert.com/post/155073242136/the-climate-science-challenge> (accessed 04.01.17).

Arnoldussen, N.T., 2016. The Social Construction of the Dutch Air Quality Clash. Boomjuridisch, Den Haag.

Biswas, A.K., Kirchherr, J. Prof, no one is reading you. *The Straits Times* April 11, 2015. See <http://www.straitstimes.com/opinion/prof-no-one-is-reading-you> (accessed 21.11.16).

Briggs, W., 2016. Uncertainty. The Soul of Modeling, Probability & Statistics. Springer, Switzerland.

Burgess, A., 2004. Cellular Phones, Public Fears, and a Culture of Precaution. Cambridge University Press, Cambridge.

Calabrese, E.J., 2015. On the origins of the linear no-threshold (LNT) dogma by means of untruths, artful dodges and blind faith. Environ. Res 142, 432–442.

Commission of the European Communities. 2001. *White Paper—strategy for a future Chemicals Policy*. Brussels.

Committee on Health Risks of Exposure to Radon (BEIR VI), 1999. *Health Effects of Exposure to Radon*. National Academy Press, Washington, DC.

Eagleton, T., 2009. Reason, Faith, and Revolution: Reflections on the God Debate. Yale University Press, New Haven, CT.

Feinstein, A., 1988. Scientific standards in epidemiologic studies of the menace of daily life. Science 242, 1257–1263.

Furedi, F., 2002. Culture of Fear. Risk-Taking and the Morality of Low Expectations. Continuum, London.

Godfrey-Smith, P., 2003. Theory and Reality. University of Chicago Press, Chicago, IL.

Hook, E.B. (Ed.), 2002. Prematurity in Scientific Discovery. On Resistance and Neglect. University of California Press, Berkeley, Los Angeles, London.

Ioannidis, J.P., 2005. Why most published research findings are false. PLoS Med. 2 (8), 696–701.

Nagel, T., 1986. The View from Nowhere. Oxford University Press, Oxford.

Newton-Smith, W.H., 1981. The Rationality of Science. Routledge, London, New York.

Pielke Jr., R., 2016. My Unhappy Life as a Climate Heretic. Wall Street J.12-02-.

Polanyi, M., 1958. Personal Knowledge. Towards a Post-Critical Philosophy. Routledge, London.

Polanyi, M., 1963. The potential theory of adsorption. Authority in science has its uses and its dangers. Science 141, 1010–1013.

Yang, K., Xing, B., 2010. Adsorption of organic compounds by carbon nanomaterials in aqueous phase: Polanyi theory and its application. Chem. Rev. 110, 5989–6008.

Chapter 9

Toxicology in Science and Society—Future Challenges

By now it should be clear what a toxic compound is. Or are you now confused, but on a higher level? If so, that is a good sign. Because every compound can display toxic properties, but it is the dose related to our physiology that makes the toxin. This entails that even our daily food can be toxic to us, yet we have achieved the ability to adapt. This is the major thread that runs through our book you have now almost finished. What remains is a short overview what we have achieved and to take a look at the challenges that lay ahead.

TOXICOLOGY: FUTURE CHALLENGES IN SCIENCE

The human body possesses an elaborate coping ability. The rich capacity to handle chemicals compounds even explains the evolutionary success of aerobic life forms. These coping mechanisms make it difficult if not impossible to describe toxic responses in absolute numbers. The estimation of toxicity is always expressed as a chance, a chance of harm. In society these chances are frequently and regrettably erroneously defined as absolute damages. The increasing complexity of our society requires that we understand the meaning of the word chance. Journalists play a crucial role in this.

Also in the science of toxicology, the meaning of a toxic response in a homeostatic physiology might be more clearly demarcated as a toxicological tipping point. Changes can occur in a resilient system until this point of no return is reached. It forms a challenge for toxicology to understand and define these tipping points. The so-called threshold of toxicological concern (TTC) might be an interesting value in this respect. The TTC indicates that the body can cope with compounds until a certain threshold dose is reached where concern arises. This TTC alludes to this tipping point and toxicology becomes more in line with the notion of chance of harm and will probably be better comprehensible for nontoxicologists.

There are signs that toxicology already develops along these lines. The so-called big-data approaches are used to map the complete physiology and to subsequently describe the influence of exogenous compounds on this physiology chart. Critics doubt whether the complexity and indeed the

Toxicology: What Everyone Should Know. DOI: http://dx.doi.org/10.1016/B978-0-12-805348-5.00009-0

flexibility of the human physiology render this a successful approach. On the other hand, optimists even state that this methodology will allow prediction of toxicological tipping points for a single individual: your own big data.

And here's the difference between big data derived from many individuals and one person. Probability does not imply cause; it could never do so. But if we could extract big data related to one person, we are not looking primarily at "averages" from many individuals (probabilities) but at mechanisms of physiology of one individual. Then, cause and effect come into view. And that is what is required to understand and tackle the tipping points from homeostasis to toxicity.

Experiments with one person ($n = 1$) would then be possible. As long as recovery of the dynamic biological system occurs fast, the resilience is abundant. When repair becomes slower a toxicological tipping point is near. Surely it forms a very attractive perspective to be able to predict with early warning systems at which stage perturbation of a biological system is such that a cellular system is no longer able to recover (Table 9.1). Indicators of resilience will undoubtedly be used to characterize our personal health status, the ability to adapt.

Unlike a drug with an expected and desired biological effect, a toxic compound can exert its effect via all kinds of perturbations. This makes it difficult to predict the toxic response of a compound.

The attentive reader noticed that we frequently used words like xenobiotic or compound or substance and not chemical as so many do. After all, all compounds can elicit a toxic response, not just man-made chemicals.

Toxicological knowledge is however focused on these man-made chemicals. They are easy to investigate because they can be purchased in pure form and in large quantities. The effects of the combination of compounds (food) remain a future challenge. Our understanding on combinatorial toxicity is scarce. This should not lead to unfounded fear and putative syndromes like "multiple chemical sensitivity" should not be advocated.

Public awareness prevails that combination of compounds offers frequently more danger than single compounds. However, just by realizing that food consumption is an ultimate form of exposure to a combination of compounds

TABLE 9.1 Why Are Xenobiotics Toxic?

Xenobiotics cause toxicity by disrupting normal cell functions "to a point of no return":
- Via binding to and damage of proteins (structural proteins like enzymes)
- Via binding to and damage of DNA (mutations)
- Via binding to and damage of lipids
- Via reaction in the cell with oxygen to form "free radicals" which damage proteins, DNA, and lipids

should be reassuring in itself. In fact, the diversification of food intake is beneficial to health, which thus points at the opposite: combinations of compounds frequently offer less danger than single compounds.

Prediction of toxic effects of compounds matures. However, in the foreseeable future, it will not be possible to sufficiently understand how chemicals are metabolized in the body from predictive computer programs and tests in cells alone. Although the improvement in analytical techniques will offer possibilities to work with minute doses in humans directly, thus skipping testing in animals.

Large epidemiological studies which frequently give rise to a lot of unrest should be conducted with more methodological rigor, similarly as in medical studies, with protocol, end points, etc. defined on forehand. The outcomes should be reported reluctantly without overstatements, keeping in mind that the smaller the effects, the less like the findings will prove to be true in the long run.

Also, we should move away from the rendition of standards in mass (milligrams, micrograms, nanograms). Rather, if anything specified needs to said on standards, the mole (Avogadro's number) should be the standard. The number of molecules gives insight into the homeostatic responses and capabilities of our physiology. Mass does not convey such information.

In 2012 Daniel Kahneman wrote the book *Thinking Fast and Slow*. Our brain works in two modes, the associative and rational mode. In toxicology, as in any other area of science, both are needed, the knowledge phase and the contemplative phase. Realization of our way of thinking can guard against toxicological judgmental glitches that can bring societal trouble.

TOXICOLOGY: FUTURE CHALLENGES IN SOCIETY

We have shown that there are two routes toward regulation: from toxicology to regulation and from legislature and regulation to toxicology. In both, toxicology plays a major role but with different functionalities. In the first one, science discovers and triggers a regulatory response to tackle the problem that arose from that discovery. In the second one, toxicology is subsidiary to the wishes and demands of the legislature. Here, the scientific work is more diffuse, as it is not always clear that toxicology is equipped to handle the legislature's demands.

The crux between both strands is academic freedom. The first drives toward discovery—the hidden structure of toxicological reality—whereas the second is driven by construction of topics that might or might not be an issue within the realm of research. As a result, the second route is far more prone to public and political drivers that have less to do with the epistemic drivers of science. Although the second route has less academic clout, the societal spin-off with respect to public reassurance has value in itself. Unrest about certain toxicological issues can have its detrimental public health effects. Toxicology is then the science of reassurance.

Risk communication is of huge societal significance to value the magnitude of the risk. Education remains of utmost importance. Some basic knowledge on how compounds interact with and on the human body and how compounds behave in the environment adds in understanding possible effects of these compounds. Science journalists are pivotal players in this respect. The public needs journalists that do not blow up small accidents to huge proportions but requires journalists that bring the touch of nuance in news. Politicians should realize that regulation by itself does not eliminate risk.

And scientists should remain seeking the academic debate. They should continue to admit that we still have limited knowledge on effects that can occur mostly in daily life, which is at a low-level exposure of compounds. That knowledge is growing, and fortunately not in a linear fashion but in much more exciting ways. We have shared a number of those exciting developments.

REFERENCES AND FURTHER READING

Hanekamp, J.C., Pieterman, R., 2009. Risk communication in precautionary culture—the precautionary coalition. Hum. Exp. Toxicol. 15 (1), 5—6.
Kahneman, D., 2012. Thinking Fast and Slow. Penguin Books Ltd.

Index

Note: Page numbers followed by "*f*" and "*t*" refer to figures and tables, respectively.